Cancer

Beating The Odds

By

Michael J. McCartney MES, MHSc.

ISBN 978-0-9683341-2-6

McCartney, Michael J. 1951-

www.Archangel-Books.com

Published by: Archangel Publications

Editor: Liz Fleming

LizArchangelPublications@gmail.com

The Author may be contacted through the Publisher or the author's website (www.michaeljmccartney.com).

Contents

Who Will Benefit From This Book

This book was written for you, if you or your friend or loved one has been diagnosed with cancer. It is also for individuals who want to help prevent cancer from occurring.

This is a practical book that will help those diagnosed with cancer to beat the odds if they follow the empowering suggestions in each chapter. This book will inform the reader about diet, lifestyle issues, stress reduction and many other factors proven to extend their lives.

The author has written this book to share what he has learned about cancer. He is a scientist, a former health care consultant and a cancer survivor. As a patient he understands what it is like to be diagnosed, to go through treatment, to be told his life will be limited by cancer. As an insider, he has used his education and insider information in his personal fight with cancer and he has turned his experiences, and research into this book to help others with cancer.

His sincere hope is that this book will help people who have been diagnosed with cancer, their families and friends as well as helping others to postpone or even prevent cancer from occurring.

There is hope, there are ways to beat the odds.

Dedication

This book is dedicated to the millions of cancer related health professionals and workers who are employed in hospitals, clinics and private settings. The majority of these individuals strive with compassion and enthusiasm to help those stricken with cancer and their families.

This book is also dedicated to one of the fathers of modern healthcare, Sir William Osler (1849-1919). He was a Canadian physician who lived and worked in the US and Britain and was known for his pithy comments and humour. Many of his sayings are as true for healthcare today as they were when he originally spoke them, too many have been forgotten. Here is one for those diagnosed with cancer to live by:

"Shut out all of your past except that which will help you weather your tomorrows."

Sir William Osler

To my wife Elizabeth who is my number one team member and love of my life, to my wonderful children, Barbara, Andrew and John. To my parents, sister Andra and friends, and last but not least to my sister Judith who was taken too early by cancer. A special thanks to the over 200 individuals who contributed their often heart wrenching stories of cancer, and last but not least to the over 30 health professionals who agreed to be interviewed for this book.

Thank you

Introduction

INTRODUCTION

"It is health that is real wealth and not pieces of gold and silver."

Mahatma Gandhi

We live in a busy world, one in which most of us take our body and health for granted, that is, until we become very ill. Then,without further ado, stopping everything else, we must deal with the hand we have been dealt.

Only when we are diagnosed with a serious illness do we begin to realize that we should have been paying more attention to maintaining our health. It is usually then and only then that we realize how precious life is, how important taking care of ourselves really is.

With this new health focussed mindset we can begin the process of gathering the knowledge we need to help us beat the odds and improve the chances of surviving our cancer diagnosis.

How To Read This Book

You don't need to be told how to read a book. That being said you need to know that although the chapters are independent of each other, the most benefit will come from reading the whole book. So, after you have read the introduction feel free to read the other chapters in what ever order you wish. Remember though that the book is a package, and every chapter deals with topics essential to your recovery.

Throughout the book we will learn interesting information from the stories of people we talked to who were diagnosed with cancer. We will learn first hand from them how to steel ourselves for dealing with cancer. Their stories cover their initial reactions to the diagnosis, the decisions you will need to consider and make, the bumps in the road of treatment, to the goal of a permanent remission, or as close to it as you can get. Their stories are an important part of this book. One story in particular has its own appendix. Allan and I have not yet met in person but we shared his journey through cancer treatment to recovery over the internet. Read appendix three if you need to be uplifted by his positive attitude and humour.

1. Chapter One is about obtaining knowledge.

A cancer diagnosis is a situation where "knowledge is power". We will discuss how to use free tools to gain knowledge such as internet healthcare sites, libraries, government agencies and other not for profit associations. The goal being to learn what experts know about your diagnosis and treatment. We will learn how to build our own database of information. A knowledgeable person with a cancer diagnosis is a much stronger individual who is more likely to beat the odds.

2. Chapter Two is about strategy.

You or your loved one has been diagnosed with cancer. What should you do? Who should you talk with? Who should you believe? How can you reduce the stress and anxiety that comes with the diagnosis? Where can you turn for help? How should you approach this challenge? We need a strategy for dealing with challenges in life, a personal strategy will empower those diagnosed with cancer. An empowered patient is empowered to beat the odds.

3. Chapter Three is about your helpers.

It is about building your team to deal more effectively with the cancer diagnosis. The suggested team goes beyond your family doctor and oncologist. We will discuss other absolutely key people who will help you to beat the odds. Depending on your background and experience you will undoubtedly have holes in your knowledge base that others can help to fill, we all do. We will discuss who can be helpful and who you need to have on your team to cover all the bases. Developing your dream team will help you to beat the odds.

4. Chapter Four will help you with your nutrition.

Food is very important, some say that 90% of some cancers (Colon, Breast and Prostate for example) are directly related to dietary issues, things like pesticides in food and trans fats. All individuals with cancer diagnoses can benefit from increasing their intake of cancer fighting foods. The evidence shows that certain foods promote cancer while other foods fight cancer. Food allergies have been theorized to affect cancer. Allergies may contribute to physiological stress and reduce the effectiveness of the immune system. The good news is that some foods fight cancer. So chapter four has suggestions on how to research and find foods that are good for you and recipes that are appealing and will help you fight cancer. You and your cancer are unique, you need to learn to create your own unique diet to fight cancer and beat the odds.

5. Chapter Five is about the importance of movement/ exercise.

Actually it is more about how to keep moving. With cancer and even some treatment options (surgery, chemotherapy and radiation therapy to name three) getting off the couch can be a chore. We discuss how and when to do this. Exercise has been shown to be a very effective way to boost the immune system and gene repair. We will discuss how to determine how much movement is appropriate for you. Also, we will discuss the types of exercise that are appropriate, how to ease into it and how to stay the course to help beat the odds.

6. Chapter Six is about treatment options.

Not only how to evaluate them but how to avoid bias from your heath care providers, and who to bring into your circle of helpers who can act as decision advisors.

Too many people have failed to beat the odds because they made bad treatment choices, this is about improving your personal decision making process to help you beat the odds.

7. Chapter Seven is about cures that occur unexpectedly.

These cures are also known as spontaneous remission, spontaneous regression or a miraculous cure. Miracles do happen. This chapter discusses spontaneous remission and how to make that a more likely event for you. There are powerful techniques that will improve your chances of attaining a complete remission. We discuss the science and the things beyond science.

8. Chapter Eight deals with stress.

The cancer diagnosis is traumatic, how we deal with our mental reaction and those of others is important for beating the odds. This chapter is about how we can improve our mental toughness. How we can reduce our reaction to negative stress. In addition we will analyze how our care team can help us. Health professionals agree on one thing, people with a cancer diagnosis who are mentally prepared will live longer than the average, they beat the odds.

9. Chapter Nine is about hope and spirituality.

Whether you are religious or not you need to know how strength of spirit and deeply felt hope can affect your likelihood of beating the odds. Beating the odds is possible and believing in your capability to fight the big fight takes courage and smart choices. Learn how to improve your inner grace to stay the course.

10. Chapter Ten is about enhancements to healthcare.

No matter where you live, what regime you live under or whether you have money or not, the way health care is provided is not ideal for cancer. Cancer cuts across many organ systems and thus many professional areas. These silos cause communications and organizational issues. We discuss how we can improve our odds by being creative within the system, knowing which buttons to push, who to call, and when to “stir the pot” to ensure individuals with a cancer diagnosis get the treatment they need when they need it.

Appendices

There are three Appendices the first contains a unifying theory for cancer, the second appendix lists resources that the author found helpful in his fight against cancer and the third appendix chronicles an individuals cancer journey through emails. The first appendix is about carcinogens, cancer types and body system function; it ties together information about cancer. A theory is proposed to help create a vision or a macro view of cancer. Understanding the whole picture will help many people see the wisdom behind the recommendations that are made in this book.

A brief introduction to this theory is essential for the reader to understand so here is a summary of what is in that appendix.

A Unifying Theory Of Cancer

There are many scholarly discussions about components of a theory that contribute to an understanding of how cancer cells grow, most require a good science background to understand. None of these components provide an overarching cancer theory. One example of these components is the current debate about whether metastasis is due to cancer cells acting like white blood cells. Another is about the purpose of telomeres. Telomeres are said to limit the life of chromosomes and when they are shortened or attacked this may lead to cancer. Such theories are a useful scholarly debate which will contribute to further cancer research "breakthroughs". The problem is that these micro theories deal with disaggregated pieces of the cancer story and they tend to be physical in nature. It is difficult for patients to "see" the whole picture.

For the record, here is the usual way that oncologists and cancer researchers explain cancer to patients and families: *"Either due to heredity, exposure to trauma or a carcinogen something transforms or alters a normal cell.*

1. A further mutation may cause a precancerous cell, then over time it may become a cancerous cell.
2. The altered genetic material in the cell sends a wrong message.
3. Often,the cell begins to divide rapidly. The cell forgets to stop dividing.

4. It forms a lump or tumour which needs to be treated.

There is a “silent” period when cancer cells are forming and multiplying where there are no associated health issues; then when a certain cell mass is reached the tumour or its effects on the body are noticeable and a diagnosis occurs. At some point in this process, screening may identify cancer before symptoms are seen.

A variation of this basic cancer theory is that we carry "Oncogenes" along with our normal genes but they aren't activated in a normal body. There is some evidence that certain genes are present before a certain cancer occurs, the problem is that they aren’t found in all cases. The oncogenes or the normal gene mutation occurs when one or more “carcinogens”, (something that activates and or mutates), hits the cell. Carcinogens are things like smoke, radiation, food contaminants, viruses, etc.”

Unifying Theory-Summary

Clearly in the common explanations above, that have been paraphrased from a number of sources, there are words like “something happens” or “often” or “may” which really means either “we don’t know what happens” or that it is too complicated to explain to laypeople.

The main problem with this way of explaining cancer is that it is too linear. The impression we are left with is that cancer happens and there is nothing you can do about it.

This is the wrong impression to give to recovering cancer patients, as we will see there is much you can do.

Here is our synthesis of the large amount of evidence we analyzed in preparing this book, for want of a better name we are calling it the ***Unifying Theory.***

As an oncologist friend said to me "Michael, to be honest, we don't know anything about cancer other than some things seem to work on some people some of the time."

He was being humble, cancer researchers actually know many things about cancer, but he was right in that there is no consistent unifying theory for cancer. This lack of a macro view of cancer is not helpful to those patients who have to wait for a cure. Our minds need to make sense of the cancer to feel in control of it, the unifying theory helps.

Hypothesis One: The development of cancer is not a linear process but a circular one.

What we mean by this is that the body is very good at fighting disease. There are many self regulating systems in the body. The body is always changing, as we change our diet, as our stress levels change, our body responds with chemical changes constantly. We know from pathologists evidence that cancer has many false starts in the body before it proliferates to a point where it is an issue. As the chemical environment in our body changes, we either fight cancer or create an environment that is conducive to cancer cell proliferation.

This “circularity” explains many things, for example; why some individuals are diagnosed then get well (spontaneous remission), and perhaps more importantly for the rest of us, why people who are diagnosed and treated beat the odds and live far beyond their doctors expectations.

Stress is more than psychological, it is also physical. Pain is an example of physical stress, but so is being chronically tired or overweight or suffering from a chronic disease like heart disease or diabetes. Even eating a poor diet can induce metabolic stress.

Physical stress has been known for a long time. In 1775 a British surgeon linked chimney soot to a form of cancer unique to chimney sweeps. He did this by observation. It wasn’t until 1918 that researchers were able to actually induce cancer on the earlobes of rabbits using tar. Carcinogens like tar and soot can trigger cancer in certain individuals. Today there are thousands of carcinogens.

Chronic diseases are a different example of physical stress. Using diabetes as an example, the diabetic person has difficultly controlling their blood sugar. Insulin is a hormone produced in the pancreas to control blood sugar. Diabetes can be caused by too little insulin production or body resistance to insulin produced or both. The blood chemistry changes causing stress. Insulin moves glucose from our blood stream to our muscles, fat and liver cells where it can be used as fuel or energy. Diabetics also develop compromised livers (fatty liver) which reduces the filtering capability of the liver. The compromised energy creation system can affect the bodies ability to fight disease. Diabetics as a result are more likely to get certain cancers. An interesting recent finding confirms that certain drugs given to diabetics to control their disease also reduce the rate of growth of certain cancer tumours. Asthmatics also have a higher incidence of cancer, as do people who are chronically depressed. Stress is a powerful force in disease.

It is well known that psychological and physical stress (pain, depression, etc.) cause specific chemicals to be released in the body. This is a natural part of the bodies self regulatory process. The problem is not the occasional chemical releases in response to daily living but the chronic exposure to these naturally occurring chemicals.

Long term depression causes parts of the brain to shrink. This is due to chemicals released in response to the disease. Some of these chemicals have now been linked to cancer. One example is adrenaline, it is released in reaction to negative stress and has been recently shown to accelerate tumor growth.

Hypothesis Two : Stress from different sources is additive and if chronic and/or sufficiently intense it can trigger cancer.

What we mean by this is that negative thinking causes stress, physical strain causes stress, exposure to carcinogens cause physical or chemical stress, trauma causes stress, these types of stress cause the body to release chemicals which causes metabolic stress. All this stress in combination helps to trigger cancer cells to proliferate. The evidence that we have missed to date is that these forms of stress are additive.

Hans Selye, the celebrated psychology researcher, proved that psychological stress was additive. Changing jobs, divorce, having an argument, etc. each adds to the stress load. Science has not yet determined a way of measuring our total stress load.

In the unifying cancer theory we take this one step further. In addition to psychological stress being additive, we theorize that psychological, metabolic, physiological and respiratory stresses are all additive. Medicine tends to separate body and mind; in the unifying theory we are arguing that they are not separate at all. Mental and physical stress are additive.

Here is an example of physical stress being additive. Over sixty years ago it was shown that half of the patients with asbestosis went on to develop lung cancer, but if the patient smoked, that percentage increased significantly. This started the idea that multiple physical hits on a gene was more likely to trigger cancer. Our view on this is that the stress was additive and it triggered immune system compromise, as well as lowered defenses which resulted in increased risk of genetic changes and the cancer.

The fact that psychological stress also contributes to cancer, is well documented. Perhaps most well known is that there is a higher rate of cancer found in holocaust survivors.

It makes sense that physical body stress is also additive. We see this in patients with multiple diseases. As a simple example, if your body is hot on a very hot day, your reaction to a minor infection is much worse. Our emergency departments become full in hot weather, respiratory ailments amplify, as do other diseases. So we see the additive nature of bodily stresses every day in healthcare.

As we are exposed to environmental stress, psychological stress, asthma, heart disease, diabetes, the stresses add up. It is very likely that one of two things is going on. First, the immune system becomes overloaded or compromised, second, the bodies ability to repair mutations to the gene sequence is affected. Recent research into telomeres for example has suggested that stress may reduce the length of telomeres, thus contributing to cancer. Telomeres are the shoe lace ends on chromosomes, telomeres protect chromosomes. Every time a chromosome divides as cells are replaced the telomeres shorten. However, the telomeres also shorten for other reasons, one reason may be stress.

Researchers tell us that gene mutations occur every day and are repaired every day in a “normal” person. The Unifying theory argues that when advancing age and/or exposure to bacteria or viruses, or toxins in food, water and air add up they cause stress to the body which creates an environment in which cancer cells can grow.

Recent research has confirmed that aerobic exercise, for example, is good stress which stimulates the body to release chemicals which form a protective gene repair function. So, some stress causes cancer to proliferate and other good stress causes it to go into remission. This occurs every day in every body. This is good evidence for the Unifying theory argument for the cyclical nature of cancer cell growth.

In terms of cancer proliferation, with increasing negative stress, the normal repair mechanisms are compromised, they cannot repair the increase in number of mutations and the result is a change either to the gene or its function. Combine this with the fact that stress compromises the immune system and we have a double impact.

With continued or chronic negative stress, cells in a particular area of the body start becoming cancerous. Instead of unhealthy cells dying normally, cancer cells proliferate and a tumour forms. If the proliferation is too advanced or cancer treatment isn't started early enough the cancer may metastasize out of the initial area, eventually leading to death unless drastic changes are made to reduce all stress.

This additive stress model explains why people living in relatively toxin free environments, who avoid foods and drinks that contain toxins, who live a relatively stress free life and are physically active have much lower incidence rates for cancer. If the same people move to a developed country with pollution, more daily stress, are exposed to toxic people, toxic food and water, and don't exercise the cancer cell proliferation is triggered at a younger age. We observe this to be a fact.

Hypothesis Three: Cancer cell proliferation is cyclical, varying according to the total stress load.

The proliferation of cancer cells may slow or stop by itself and not proceed. We know this because many autopsies reveal a presence of undiagnosed cancer, unrelated to cause of death. In these situations we theorize that either stress was low level and so the cancer was kept relatively under control by the body and lifestyle or that at some point the cancer promoting stress peaked and then dropped back to lower levels, causing the cancer to recede.

The other evidence of this is the scientifically documented phenomenon of spontaneous remission. Cancer is diagnosed, the patient puts their life on hold, goes for treatment (that is not expected to "cure" the cancer), then something unexpected happens and the cancer goes away for a while or for ever.

This part of the theory is key to beating the odds. If you get diagnosed, immediately start reducing all the negative psychological, physiological and other negative stress from your life. This book will help with that.

Hypothesis Four: In cases where no cure is known, standard medical treatment is not enough.

While this sounds like an obvious statement, many patients and health professionals don't act as though it is. Classical medical treatment often involves chemical targeting of the cancer, radiation of the cancer or removal of the tumor by surgery. If all the affected cells are removed this may be successful.

The issue that this theory underlines is that all the cancer cells may not die and the cancer may return if the treatment did not get all the cancer cells. This is much more liable to happen if you continue to live the way you did before the treatment. You will be better off and have a better chance of beating the odds if you reduce your negative stress load in addition to having medical treatment. This may involve lifestyle changes including diet, exercise, meditation, counseling, as well as complementary and alternative treatments in addition to the medical treatment. The remainder of this book is about empowering you to make those changes in your life.

Beating The Average

This book is a self help manual to help you extend your life. It is firmly based on scientific research and the experiences of individuals who have extended their lives beyond the time medical advice expected.

This is very important to remember. When a health professional or the internet or a relative tells you that people with your diagnosis have a finite number of weeks, months or years to live, you need to understand something key, something that is fundamental to science. Scientific predictions are based on statistics from the past being projected forward into the future, in this case,your future.

There are two issues with this;

First, the past is not the future. A decade ago for example, few people knew about Vitamin D, today, many people take it as a daily supplement. Recent research indicates that Vitamin D may effectively reduce the progression of certain cancers. This is just one example of the many changes that have occurred in recent years.

The change in consumer behaviour, such as taking vitamin D, may have a significant effect on longevity but the statistical evidence of this won't become apparent for several years. There are many improvements to individual lifestyles like this that will make past statistics unreliable as the basis for future projection purposes.

Second, the statistics about prognosis are based on averages, here are some examples. My 90+ year old friend Bill, who has outlived his doctors was told he had two years to live 25 years ago. He beat the odds. Eva on the other hand heard she had cancer and gave up, she died well before the doctors had predicted her death to be. Paul was told he had two years to live and stopped doing anything that might help his longevity, he overindulged, went back to smoking and died sooner than expected. Those individuals were part of the statistics that created the average life expectancy following those diagnoses. Bill significantly beat the average, Eva and Paul did not.

The bottom line is that the average is an artificial number useful in studying disease in the macro sense but useless in projecting how long you will live.

You can beat the average, you can beat the odds.

The Author's Experience

Michael's cancer death sentence was pronounced when he was diagnosed. According to the powers that be, Michael was to die two years after diagnosis. He was told he was palliative. The author was asked whether he wanted to bother with treatment. He was 58 years old.

Hopefully you will not have a similar experience, to put it lightly, that was not the best day Michael had ever had!

To top it off, that same month he found out that his younger sister's cancer had returned, she was terminal, she died two months later at the age of 47. Not the best year of the McCartney families life either!

We started this book two years and one month after the author's diagnosis. By that time Michael and the team he had assembled to help beat the odds had been working hard to thwart the medical prognosis and extend his life using many methods. This was accomplished by researching all the diverse methods that fight cancer and following everything suggested in this book. The unifying theory came out of this work. The strategies that were evidence based and passed muster were put into effect, Michael's life changed accordingly.

As the research paid off for Michael he wanted to document what we had found so that others might also benefit. So this is not a treatise by a researcher who never had cancer, or a parent or spouse or friend or relative of someone who had cancer. This book was written because Michael was diagnosed with cancer and has lived through the cancer treatment system, so to use the vernacular, Michael is "walking the walk and talking the talk".

The author's academic credentials were very helpful in understanding the science, being a health care insider certainly helped, but the actual cancer diagnosis and treatment experience was the catalyst for this book. There is more about the author on page 303.

To beat the odds we used our investigative skills, analytical skills and inside knowledge as health professionals and scientists.

Our conclusion;

We can assure you that there are ways to beat the odds.

Let me repeat that in another way;

"There is scientific evidence that we can beat the odds and extend our lives beyond the average life expectancy for most cancers."

What you need to do is read this book and do what is recommended in each and every chapter. The book is written to "teach you to fish", as the saying goes.

The Cancer Epidemic

The cancer epidemic globally was recently documented as costing over $290 billion per year for new cases and increasing annually. The 13 million new cases per year in 2009 is expected to increase to 17 million new cases per year by 2020. The cancer burden on society globally has doubled in the last 30 years. Cancer now accounts for 20% of all deaths annually.

According to the Cancer Society one in two men and one in three women will be afflicted by cancer in their lives. The global incidence is anticipated to go from one in three to one in two by 2015.

One reason that cancer has become a leading cause of death is that health science has invented treatments for so many of the diseases that used to kill people before they could get cancer. Cancer used to be more often a disease of the elderly. However in the US cancer is also the number 2 killer of children aged 1 to 14. Having money helps, low income individuals with cancer are more likely to die than high income individuals (75% vs 46%). Individuals who live in developed countries are more likely to die of cancer than those from less developed countries (where infectious and other diseases have not yet been beaten).

Cancer is a word that strikes fear into the heart of every sane person. We don't understand it, for the most part, we can't cure it. We usually can't see it. In addition most individuals don't really know where it comes from, why it suddenly starts or why it goes into "remission".

We often hear that we really don't know very much about cancer at all given the large fortune that has been spent on researching it since the "war on cancer " was declared in

1971. Current estimates are that over $20 Billion is spent on cancer research annually. There are many brilliant minds who have spent a large part of their lives trying to understand cancer. We respect their work and their dedication and believe that they will succeed eventually.

The problem is, what do those of us who have been diagnosed with incurable cancer do in the interim?

This book is about what we can do until effective cures have been created. We are not suggesting that you abandon traditional scientific approaches to treatment, we are suggesting you supplement medical treatment and become an active participant in your care making serious life changes that can help you beat the odds. So please give serious consideration to the information in this book.

In our interviews of over 200 individuals diagnosed with cancer we have learned that people believe that their lives are being cut short by this "unknown entity". Individuals asked for more certainty, they want to understand how to act to try to bring the cancer under control or postpone its recurrence. In short the individuals we spoke to wanted a resource book to help them to beat the odds.

Throughout the book you will find a sampling of stories recounted by the 200 individuals we interviewed or asked to tell their stories. They will look like this.....

"My friends father, Joseph worked for a major electrical component builder. His work involved building switches and electrical gears and back 30-40 years ago they used lots of PCB's and other chemicals now known to be toxic. When he was diagnosed with cancer a few years ago both he and his family tried to get the health professionals to record that he worked in the electrical industry and was exposed to toxic materials but their eyes glazed over. To my knowledge nobody documented the exposure to toxic chemicals which is most probably the cause of his cancer since a lot of his coworkers also died of cancer".

This story illustrates a healthcare system issue which needs correction to assist in the fight against cancer. Many health system issues are discussed in chapter ten.

Most of the stories from those we interviewed are used, to illustrate points that are important to learn from. An exception is the long story in appendix three, included to give the reader an entertaining but important insight into one person's journey from diagnosis, to treatment, to recovery.

Complementary And Alternative Approaches

The majority of cancer patients get their main care through medically focussed health systems. This will result in them having an average outcome. If we aren't satisfied with an average outcome, we need to keep an open mind, about the issues in this book. Beating the odds requires thinking outside the box and becoming an active participant in our healthcare recovery. This means we need to explore alternative and complementary options as well as medical options. The question is, how can we do this safely?

It is frustrating that the successes of many alternative methods are often inconsistent. They work well with some people but not with others. The lack of consistency is of concern, replicability is a cornerstone of the scientific method. The major question is that since some alternative approaches do work with some people, not all, does that necessarily negate using the approaches? This is where strict evidence based approaches to health treatment takes a very rigid view that may be very shortsighted. In some cases we may be throwing the baby out with the bathwater.

Those individuals who write off alternatives as being nothing but a placebo may be simplistic in their thinking. The evidence is much stronger and we will discuss how science may need to rethink how to study such cases. This is important for the person with the cancer diagnosis to comprehend, because how you interpret the information will directly affect your ability to beat the odds.

So our approach in this book is from two angles, the classical medical and the alternative and complementary, within reason....

Quacks And Scam Artists

On the other side of the coin, we have all heard the salesman who tells you he was diagnosed with colon cancer and cured himself by inventing a juice drink he can sell to you for only $20, (if you act now you can get 2 for $20!). They present no evidence and a lot of hype. This book is not about that. This book is about beating the odds with scientific evidence that relies on evidence based research, and applying common sense. We will not be suggesting unproven methods. We will discuss how to identify scams.

Being Careful

Information is everywhere, in newspapers, in scientific journals, magazines and on the internet. What should you believe? Reporters vary in their ability to interpret medical findings, some health reporters are very knowledgeable and can be relied upon, but others cover health as a sideline and sometimes make some grand blunders. It is best to go to the research source to understand what is being reported.

Follow the internet search advice in chapter one to find scientific information you can rely on.

The Middle Way

As mentioned, the cancer patient's best interests are not always served by the norm in health care, the status quo can be flawed.

Sometimes a combination of "alternative" and status quo methods are better.

Jeff tells us " When I was having radiation therapy, the daily radiation knocked the good bacteria out of my gut. This caused a stomach upset and made certain foods unpalatable since they became indigestible.

A member of my personal health team, my naturopathic doctor suggested I take a dose of a probiotic bacteria every day after radiation. There was scientific evidence, that it would not interfere with the radiation treatment, and was effective, so I took it. That stopped my indigestion.

Not being disturbed by the indigestion really helped my sense of well being during this difficult time. The medical team on the other hand had recommended a drug solution that simply acted on the symptoms instead of curing the underlying problem (i.e. the lack of bacteria).

This latter treatment, the drug solution prescribed by the medical team actually made me worse due to side effects, so I stopped taking it and went with the naturopathic recommendation which was the non-mainstream "common sense" solution.

Later, when I was sitting in the waiting room, waiting for radiation, other patients complained of horrible indigestion, they were losing weight, losing their will to fight. Keep in mind, that the radiation weakens the individual, so after a few weeks of radiation and little food due to digestive problems, the impact is quite profound, this is not just a mild stomach upset.

So I told the other radiation patients of the natural non-drug solution and they copied it to good effect. They regained weight, and their attitude became more positive."

This is a simple but good example of a situation where patients would benefit from a broader healthcare team than the one that is normally provided within health systems. Further, the patient's benefited from the use of non-patentable healthcare products.

My Urologist referred me to the College of Naturopathic Medicine's cancer clinic before my radiation treatment started. My experience has been a good one, see chapter three for other team building suggestions.

The main lesson from Jeff's story is that we all must be aware that we will not necessarily get the best care by leaving the responsibility to others. Wonderful as they are they work in a system that rewards certain behaviours and punishes others. The health care culture has unwritten rules that don't always work in the best way for all patients.

The result is;

We must assume some degree of responsibility for our own care!

Cancer Basics

To take responsibility we need a basic amount of knowledge about cancer jargon. Being diagnosed with cancer will expose you to medical words you are not familiar with. Latin was originally used on the premise that it was more precise. It is, and so it should be used between health professionals who are discussing healthcare issues. It should ***not*** be used when health professionals communicate with patients.

There is a culture shift occurring in healthcare. Today there is an expectation that the health professions will help patients make informed decisions about their healthcare. The use of medical jargon is not considered helpful to patients.

One sad consequence of confusing patients by using Latin and science terms is that many patients give up trying to understand their condition and their treatment and abdicate their responsibility to be the master of their own destiny to doctors and other health professionals. As we saw from many of the stories we collected, this is not always a good idea. The following explanation will be helpful.

It is important that you understand the basic words and concepts introduced here since our whole team needs to be on the same page. Along with the unifying theory, these concepts and words are some of the building blocks you need to understand cancer and have it clear in your mind.

Cancer is a set of diseases caused by out-of-control cell growth. Each type of cancer (there are well over 100) is ***classified*** by the type of cell initially affected (e.g. breast cancer). This can be confusing if the cancer returns and affects another area of the body, but this is the naming convention currently used.

Cancer causes damage to the body when cells divide uncontrollably to form lumps of tissue called ***tumours***.

Leukemia is an exception where normal blood function is disturbed by abnormal cell division.

Cancerous tumours can interfere with the body systems, causing various negative effects. Tumours that grow and are malignant are cancerous, tumours that are not malignant are ***benign***. Benign tumours don't metastasize.

Two things may be associated with cancer growth:

1. Cancer can move throughout the body using the blood or lymph systems. ***Invasion*** of another part of the body by the cancer is called ***metastasis.***

2. Cancer cells may divide and grow into a tumour, making new blood vessels to feed itself in a process called ***angiogenesis***.

So put simply, various cancer treatments (including supplements and cancer fighting foods) either stop the cancer making new blood vessels, stop it from invading other cells or slow the growth. New designer drugs and vaccines are being developed to target the different forms of cancer.

Until designer drugs exist for all cancers, the most common existing methods of fighting cancer are, radiation, chemotherapy and/or surgery these essentially remove or kill the cancer cells or create an environment cancer can no longer live in.

Cancer Causes - Certain parasites, viruses and bacteria increase the chances of getting certain cancers (e.g. Human Papilloma Virus(HPV) has been linked to the development of cervical cancer)are these stressors or triggers?Exposure to toxins like asbestos and cigarette smoke have been linked to the development of lung cancer. Heredity plays a role in some cancers for example breast cancer can run in families. Negative stress weakens the immune system and can influence your ability to fight cancer. See Appendix one for a more lengthy version of the unified model of cancer mentioned earlier in this introduction.

Caregivers

There are a wide variety of qualified individuals who may play an active role in your treatment, here are the professionals you are more likely to encounter.

- ***Oncologists*** are researchers and medical clinicians specializing in the prevention, study, diagnosis, and treatment, of cancer.
- ***Nurses*** are trained to various levels and will have different roles on your health care team. Nurse Practitioners are highly trained close to the level of physicians and they can often perform roles that once were designated solely to physicians like ordering diagnostic tests and prescribing basic pharmaceuticals. Registered Nurses are trained to monitor and treat patients but they do not have authority to order tests or prescribe medical treatments on their own initiative.
- ***Naturopaths*** are holistic doctors who use ***alternative and complementary*** approaches to treatment. In some jurisdictions they are part of the team, but more usually

they are separate. They may be contacted individually or via a college of naturopathy.

- ***Nutritionists/ Dietitians and Nutritional counsellors*** are trained in the impact of food on health, they can suggest foods known to fight cancer.
- ***Psychologists/ Psychiatrists*** help us to understand how our mind is affected by a cancer diagnosis. They can help with the mind over matter component of cancer.
- Many other specialists may be involved in your care, if you have a good ***Family Practitioner or family health team*** they will often help to monitor indicators of success and explain why the other specialists are needed and what their role is.

Alternative and complementary treatments are those not usually used by licensed medical practitioners. Depending on your diagnosis this may involve use of certain supplements, or such practices as acupuncture which can reduce pain in some individuals.

Chemotherapy is the use of drugs to treat cancer. Drugs usually have ***side effects***, that may harm you in some way. The side effects are tolerated because the the drug will extend your life, so it is a trade off situation. You need to inform yourself of the side effects, sometimes they don't appear for a while.

Jill was diagnosed with anemia, it was not listed as a side effect of the drug treatment she was receiving. She began treatment, then when she became anemic she asked her oncologist. The oncologist said that anemia was a known side effect of the drug she was given, even though the drug company didn't list it in the side effects provided by Jill's pharmacy. They listed fatigue, we can be fatigued without having anemia! The side effects of the drug treatment were severe, but after discussing the pro's and cons with her team she decided that it was not severe enough for her to stop taking the drugs."

Research

Now we understand the basic terminology, a few words on research. Most Oncologists will argue that the only research worth following is "***peer reviewed, double blind clinical research",*** quite a mouthful. This is considered the "gold standard" of clinical research. The best studies from a scientific perspective are double or triple blind studies. In this type of experiment, the researcher doesn't know which patient is getting the treatment and which are getting placebos. Peer reviewed means that an unrelated expert in that field has reviewed the methods and results used and has approved of them.

There is no doubt in my mind that this research is rock solid. In an ideal world such extensive evidence based research would be the only way to go.

That being said however, it is interesting that much of what is practiced by licensed physicians today has been handed down over the years in medical schools and has not undergone the rigor of peer reviewed double blind clinical research. This is because it is very expensive.

When it comes to cancer , due to the relatively recent nature of the research we see considerably more peer reviewed work being used to support the pharmaceutical industry drugs that are being used.

Another reason this published work is the "gold standard" is because other scientists with the same specialty have reviewed it, it is thus open to criticism.

Non-peer reviewed information is more suspect, sometimes unfairly.

Naturopaths, nutritionists and medical doctors use a mixture of peer reviewed and non-peer reviewed information in their practices. It is the non-peer reviewed information that is most subject to disagreement between the different disciplines, often due to the fact that the rigors of science are not as apparent.

Questioning The Scientific Method

The basic disagreement around the evaluation of clinical research stems from the scientific method.

The history of the scientific method is interesting, it has evolved over time from simple trial and error to a very complex set of rules. It is quite rigorous, especially when humans are being used in the experiments. We need to be thankful of that.

Research Process

Generally when applied to health care research involves:

- Measurement of data, for example, the number of people with ovarian cancer who had been treated with drug x and went into remission.
- Testing a hypothesis, for example, drug x extends the life of test subjects compared with those on a placebo.
- Patients must be comparable, that is, they are part of a clearly defined group. An example of a clearly defined group would be females from the ages of 25 to 35 with ovarian cancer that has not metastasized.
- Patients and researchers must not know who is getting the treatment and who is getting the placebo, this is the double blind aspect.
- It must be a repeatable experiment, another researcher doing the same experiment should get the same results, this is the rule of replicability.

On this last point, if you remember the big cold fusion experiment announcement a few years ago, cold fusion was going to solve the energy crisis. Their problem was that nobody else could repeat the experiment, so it failed the scientific method test of replicability.

Clinical Trials

So what does this have to do with beating the odds with cancer? The main criticism of the scientific method as applied to clinical research is that it is very expensive. A study in the New England Journal of Medicine estimated that it costs about $100 million on average to bring a drug to market. Drug companies have argued it costs much more, in some cases up to $2 billion per drug. This is beyond the reach of most small corporations, universities, foundations and individuals.

The result is that promising alternatives which cannot be patented or will not generate a profit are not researched using the full "gold standard" method because of the cost.

In todays medicine the main group that can afford to practice gold standard clinical research are the large corporations that will benefit from the results of the research.

The financial cost of the clinical trials makes it necessary that a profit results from the research. This means that in recent decades we have ended up with a large number of patentable drug based solutions in the medical field and very few other new treatments that have been tested using this extremely expensive research method and process.

Clinical trials are very expensive because of the long process that has to be used; here is a short overview of the process.

- Initially, drugs are created in the lab and tested, then after consideration of these results they are tested on animals.
- After trials on animals have shown promising results, human trials may be approved. First one has to prove that the product won't kill healthy people, and also document what the side effects are.
- Next one has to test the drug on patients with the disease, the goal being to actually prove that it helps treat the disease better than current medical practices.
- This is done in small trials first then larger trials.
- "Blind" studies are used to ensure that the researcher interacting with the patient does not know who is getting the drug and who is getting the ***placebo.***

A placebo is usually an "inert" substance given in place of the drug being tested. The placebo effect is when patients report improvements or side effects from these inert substances. In one study healthy patients given a placebo reported side effects, such as a headache, 19% of the time. Since the placebo had "side effects" another placebo may need to be used. In a recent controversial drug research study critics actually claimed that the placebo had a negative effect on the test subjects and increased deaths in that group thus making the drug look even better.

The drug has to out perform the placebo. In an ideal world it would also have to out perform current treatments and any non-patentable alternatives.

This lengthy and expensive drug test process is good for patients who benefit from the well tested drugs. There are many examples of almost miraculous results and of certain diseases disappearing from the face of the earth due to the application of such drugs. This is the great contribution of the scientific method, to our health and one that we should be very proud of. It needs to be noted however that in some cases the drugs that come out of this lengthy and expensive process are only marginally effective. One recent drug approved by the FDA only extended lives on average 4 months and cost over $100,000 per dose.

It is even more unfortunate that we are not testing the non-patentable solutions. Those alternatives that don't create a profit because they cannot be patented. A consequence of this inaction is that health system costs are increasing dramatically because potentially effective but less expensive health care alternatives are being ignored.

Why This Is Important To You

A clinical trial takes a long time to complete. It can be very frustrating if you hear in the media about a test that involved a petri dish in the lab, or on animals that sounded very positive. Everyone with the disease gets excited about a cure. Then we find out it will be years before human trials are complete. Or worse that the promising drug failed to make it through the next stage of clinical trials. That is the nature of the strict adherence to the scientific method.

Cancer sufferers with a diagnosis that has no obvious cure deserve better information about alternatives that are not patentable or profitable that can be used to extend life until "cures" are available.

The Dilemma

So how do we deal with the "other" treatments that are seen in journal articles and on the internet. Those products and services that have not been tested as rigorously? This is the dilemma.

We know that some of the "other" products and services may simply be victims of the "no patent, no profit, no research" situation. Yet again, they may simply be the product of scam artists trying to take advantage of cancer sufferers.

As cancer patients who want to beat the odds we need to clearly understand that medicine has become distorted by the "no patent, no profit, no research" approach. As a consequence, we need to consider why it is prudent to keep an open mind about safe alternatives that might be as good or even better than those from the medical industrial complex. That said, we need to be cautious. This is discussed in chapter one.

CHAPTER ONE - Knowledge Is Power

One of my medical professor colleagues talks about his medical school lectures as "his lies". He says this because he works in a field where new research happens very frequently and often the older theories he had taught become invalid, so he calls them his lies.

Research is evolving quickly and we need to be able to stay on top of it.

Good information can help us to beat the odds.

There is a very fine line between good information and misleading misinformation. We need to be able to discern between information that will help us beat the odds and misinformation that will not. There are many ways that information can be misleading.

Here is a classic example from statistics;

"***Everyone who eats a tomato will die***".

This statement is true because everybody will die sometime whether they eat a tomato or not. The point is that this statement doesn't necessarily mean that tomatoes are dangerous. This simple example illustrates that we have to be very careful to ask the right questions.

Salespeople have a way of determining what to say that will lead you to conclude that their product is the one for you to buy. They may use questionable statistics and misinformation. The tobacco industry spin doctors did this for years.

The internet is full of easy to fall into traps, the misleading sites fall into three categories. Some sites are written by well meaning foolish people, some by well meaning but greedy people and some by people with no conscience at all who are simply aiming to benefit from your misfortune.

Individuals are taken in by health misinformation due to a wide variety of reasons. Many simply lack the education to analyze the information being presented or they have a strong desire to believe in a silver bullet cure. Their desire to believe is borne out of sheer desperation. Others are misled by media coverage that is incorrect, or even by reputable researchers who just got it wrong.

So where and who should you go to for information?

There is very good information that will actually help you to beat the odds. Our task in this chapter is to learn where to go to get it.

A first place to start is the not for profit organizations that specialize in the form of cancer you have been diagnosed with. Most are run by well intentioned individuals who have a genuine desire to help and often have volunteers who are happy to help. They may also have experts who volunteer and help ensure the quality of information these agencies provide.

Some of the “not for profit” organizations have unfortunately fallen into the trap of being supported by drug companies and other corporations who benefit from cancer. While much of the information from these organizations is good, often they are loathe to criticize, that is, bite the hands that feed them. The American Cancer Society for example has been criticized from some quarters for taking large donations from the pharmaceutical industry. Follow the money trail, check them out on the internet and make sure the information they provide is without bias. Check the information out using the methods we outline in this chapter.

In 1892 many hotel rooms became equipped with electrical light, an innovation. The following notice was posted in some of the rooms:

"The room is equipped with Edison Electric Light, it is in no way harmful to your health, nor does it affect the soundness of sleep".

What Edison was referring to was that his system was direct current and he wanted to communicate to the patron that there was a risk associated with his competitors product. Unlike his competitors alternating current he claimed that his direct current would not cause electrocution. Apparently this was perceived as a huge issue before electrical standards were created.

With regards to his statement that "Edison Light is in no way harmful to your health", had any healthcare studies been done on the health effects of his system? No, he was making an unproven claim. This was a "public service announcement" to promote a product, the Edison Light. This same type of misinformation is used today by promoters of untested health products and cancer "cures".

Clearly all we are saying is be cautious until you have proof.

Continuing our search for good information, in addition to volunteer organizations, there are some government agencies that publish excellent information. On the whole they are good to excellent sources of information. That being said, lobbying is rife in governments and again, the bureaucrats must answer to politicians who rely on donations from corporations to get elected. So, it depends on the government, the strength of the government service (i.e. its ability to resist political interference) and whether they actually have the staff in place to evaluate health products and services. Government cutbacks in recent years in all western democracies have created issues. Some governments have been forced by the cutbacks to accept the word of other countries rather than doing research themselves.

Staying with the electricity example, the health effects from transmission corridors, transformers and even electrical blankets is still very controversial. Many of the research papers that said there are no effects of electricity transmission were supported by an industry group. Opponents say that industry financed researchers who come up with results that the industry doesn't like, are not financed again. This leads us to conclude...

Some Researchers Can Be influenced

A 2011 study from the Centre for Ethics at Harvard University found that no researchers funded by industry found a positive correlation between anti-depressant drugs and breast cancer but independent researchers did find a correlation. The ethics researcher was quoted as saying:

"Close industry ties can have a "pernicious" effect on the attitudes and actions of doctors and scientists. Researchers might not be aware of the subtle ways they can be influenced".

A recent investigative report by the program 60 Minutes claimed that a researcher in a major teaching centre in the US actually faked data in a cancer research study and that it may be the largest medical fraud in US history.

That being said, such unethical research is relatively rare in top tier medical journals, but follow the money.

Defining A Method That Will Work

Even as a biologist and health scientist with many years experience, including training in epidemiology and healthcare statistics, my early searches for alternative ways to slow the progression of cancer often resulted in believing information that upon more research, was later proven to be misinformation.

"One thing Jeff noted was the desperation that developed when health professionals classified me as a "terminal, palliative" cancer patient. It made my mind want to grasp at anything that might help."

If you are in the same boat, watch how your mind will grasp at straws, then resolve to follow a research path that is not based on desperation. Beating the odds takes self discipline.

So what is the best way to source good information?

Until illness intervened, the main business that the Author and his wife Elizabeth worked at was health consulting and health information research. The information they studied and analyzed extended from clinical data (e.g., how many women who had gynecological surgery ended up with adhesions) to financial information, such as "how much does a liver transplant actually cost?", and answering questions like "how can we reduce waste and save money to help more patients?"

The work gave us great insight into ways that could improve care delivery and how resources could be better allocated. One of the challenges often faced was researching a clinical issue in all its facets so that when we helped the health care organizations we could advise them about the best possible alternative. To do this we looked at other parts of the world, other ways of solving the same issues and we learned how to quickly and effectively get the best information. We became quite good at thinking "outside the box".

The author has applied this same set of techniques to the question of "beating the odds" for those diagnosed with cancer. Here is the basic information search technique.

Information Strategy

First, you need to assess your capability to judge the quality of information you are getting. Do you understand the science, the use of latin, the statistics and complex analyses? Don't worry, while you need to know the basic information we covered in the introduction, this approach will enable you to judge the quality of the information without having to earn advanced academic degrees in several fields of medicine. To start all you need is patience and a good online medical dictionary. Please refer to Appendix two the resource section for our suggested online dictionary.

Peer Review

As mentioned in the introduction, the gold standard in medical research publications is the peer reviewed research paper. To claim that your clinical research is peer reviewed means that your paper has been reviewed by a qualified researcher in the same field. Organizations like the National Institutes of Health in the US have strict guidelines for qualifying such reviewers and the review process.

In general peer reviewed medical articles, in top journals can be relied on to provide good information. So where can the lay person find such information?

One of the best free sources is a wonderful website run by the National Library of Medicine and National Institutes of Health in the US. This site is called “PubMed”.

Another great source is the UK National Institute for Health and Clinical Evidence (NICE), their portal has many excellent search capabilities. Appendix two has other suggestions for free clinical information available through the internet.

Online Search Example

For purposes of illustration we will use the Pubmed website.

Go online using Pubmed (see the link in Appendix 2, Resource section) and become familiar with the search engine.

A search on Pubmed using the search word “cancer” in 2011 for example revealed over 2.5 million articles. So we immediately have another issue, the volume of articles available. Your doctor has not read all of these, and neither can you. So your first task is to reduce the number of articles to the relevant ones by filtering. The way to start is to decide on key words to get to the articles relevant to your specific diagnosis. Key words are something of an acquired art but bear with us as we explain the process and provide some tips.

Inputting the key words “breast cancer” for example cuts down the list to almost 250,000 articles, still too large a volume. Further key words like soy cuts it down to just over 600 articles. Type in "soy and breast cancer survival", this reduces the list to a more manageable 40 articles.

The key words you use and the way they are combined will save you many hours of research, so it is worth spending some time developing your searching skill. One way to get ideas for key words is to search more generally using a search engine such as Google. For example, try putting in a question in google, like "what foods are good for breast cancer?" This yields about 130 million internet sites. Take some key words off these sites then feed them into Pubmed to see what the scholarly articles say. Spices are often mentioned in the Google search so plug in spices and breast cancer. The day we did this search we ended up with 17 articles to review.

Going back to soy and breast cancer, the forty articles we have ended up with may be organized by most recent date. If that is not how the data is presented, set the filter to arrange the articles in this manner. This is important since theories evolve over time and we want to see the most recent articles first.

The settings are adjustable. My preference is to look at the Abstract, since one can usually jump to the last couple of lines and quickly see their conclusions. This reduces the 40 articles to about 80 lines of reading. If it is very relevant I might ask for the entire paper.

Proceeding with our search of the 40 articles what information will the search uncover. One of the papers is listed as CMAJ, 2010 Nov 23:182 which means the Canadian Medical Association Journal November 23, 2010 page 182. If you want to see the entire article you can use this information to order it from a library or an online provider or the Canadian Medical Association Journal website.

Alternatively, you may wish to contact one of the authors, for example in this article Kang X is underlined so that you can click on the name and see all other articles by that author. This is a good way of focussing on their research quickly and easily. Underneath the authors names is the university or organization getting credit for their research. Here again, you will want to see if that University or organization has credibility. The classic way of doing this is to see if the University is listed in the top medical schools. Look for other journal articles and papers that have replicated the work and come to similar conclusions. To contact the author go to the University website and see if you can find an email address. Universities like to boast about their researchers and usually list their contact information.

Your doctors will most likely have read the articles from the top medical schools. Here is a list of the top medical schools from an internet search engine of the top ten in the world. The list will vary on the criteria they are judged by but this list is pretty good.

1. Harvard University

2. University of Cambridge

3. Johns Hopkins University

4. University of Pennsylvania

5. University of Oxford

6. University of California at San Francisco

7. Yale University

8. The Karolinska Institute

9. Columbia University

10. University of Dundee

My bias was to include my Alma Mater, the University of Toronto Medical School, but in this list it was ranked twelfth. Incidentally, there are over 2,200 accredited medical schools world wide, so you can understand why research from number 2,199 on the list may be less than stellar.

Consistency

So out of the forty articles you are probably interested initially in the most recent ten. Look at the conclusions, how many are consistent or is there a large amount of variability in the conclusions? If there is a large amount of consistency we can feel reasonably confident that we can believe in and act upon the information.

This all sounds like a very long involved process, in actual fact it took under an hour, with todays wi-fi and a laptop computer, to complete this task so you could do this over lunch.

The research you do is essentially doing your due diligence to ensure you have the information needed to ask the right questions and decide whether you need a second opinion or additional help in determining your personal health care plan. It is a very important process, and you need to invest the time required to do this, or get a friend or relative to help if you are not as energetic as you once were. Try asking a geek, they love this kind of thing.

There is a huge benefit to this process, with it you can feel very confident that you are doing the right thing for your diagnosis. This certainty will help to reduce your stress levels. Knowledge really is power. In addition to arming you with information so you can ask questions of your medical team, it provides you with the knowledge to confirm or deny claims being made by the “snake oil” salespeople who want you to waste your financial resources by spending your money on questionable products.

There is another even more interesting and empowering outcome of becoming an “expert” you will become a participant in determining your own path and you will often know more details about your diagnosis than many of your doctors and other health professionals. This will empower you to discuss and even when appropriate, challenge suggested treatment options.

To be fair, the reason you may know more than your health team if you stay on top of the information is that they have a wide variety of diagnoses to treat and the sheer volume of research articles makes it virtually impossible for any one person to stay on top of it all. You have only one diagnosis so you have far less information to review.

Fatal Flaw In Updating Services

My medical research friends tell me that there are now several companies offering practicing physicians an update service. For about $500 per year health professionals will be provided with frequent research updates taken from the most respectable journals by someone who has experience in the field. This is very helpful and ensures that they are on top of the latest information in their field.

This system is very useful but has its flaws. Not all the relevant research comes from “reputable” journals, top researchers and top universities because of a fatal flaw in the use of the scientific method.

Even specialists such as oncologists will miss key information if it is **not** provided by their updating internet service. Updating services focus on top universities and top researchers. Obviously, because of this they will not be aware of anything innovative that comes from allied health professions or others in the field. Clearly the top researchers in the field are the first we all want to be familiar with, but it means that the research by up and coming researchers who get their start in less prestigious universities, is often missed. Remember Einstein started in a relatively unknown

University and his early work was not as professional as his later work but still very interesting.

The "Other-Side" Of The Coin

In our search for methods to beat the odds we do not want to make the same error as the updating services. We need to consider the journals that your doctors and specialists won't read. They are either missed because they are not top tier, ignored because the content wasn't considered mainstream, and/or passed over because it was not considered "reputable".

The area of meditation provides a good example of opportunities that were missed. For many years the authors passion was trying to understand the science of meditation. This involved a twenty year search for any articles or scholarly studies relating to the science of meditation.

In the beginning pickings were slim and no "reputable" peer reviewed articles existed. To try to understand why there was no "reputable" research a number of health care experts were interviewed. These were medical researchers in fields that preliminary studies suggested meditation would benefit. This included fields such as hypertension, stress management, depression and chronic pain.

The message coming from the researchers was consistent and very clear. It was one that the author had not come across before. "We are told that meditation is not a proven method". The inference was that meditation was not effective. This flew in the face of what the preliminary research had shown. The author found this confusing since his personal experience had been very different. As a result his own research intensified.

His research revealed that the reality was quite different from what the medical researchers were saying at that time. ***The real reason was that definitive research had not been undertaken.*** There is a huge difference between "meditation is not a proven method" and the reality that the research hadn't been done.

So, who were these people who were saying that meditation was unproven? The real situation was one of: "no patent, no profit, no research". Meditation was not a patentable product or service so major corporation would benefit financially from the research.

The money trail indicated that the beneficiaries of meditation research were the individual meditation teachers and perhaps a few small organizations who offered meditation classes. The problem was that no major "for profit" corporations that normally fund healthcare research would benefit. In fact, if proven effective, meditation could affect drug company revenues when drugs were replaced by meditation. The medical industrial complex would benefit if everyone believed that "meditation was not a proven method" rather than the research hadn't been done.

Sources of research funds that are not patent related come from not for profit foundations, governments and private donors. The number of sources for non-profit research funds is much less than the for profit sector. The financial resources available are limited.

So continuing the story, in 1999 the authors first book on meditation was published, it contained a summary of the research to date and suggestions for further research. Many other individuals like Michael were also pushing at that time and recommending more evidence based meditation research. After this groundswell of interest, Government and not for profit funders began funding meditation research.

Non-Patentable But Effective

In the specific case of meditation the more advanced research confirmed the earlier supposedly “non-reputable” research. Meditation was shown to be very effective and inexpensive with no side effects. Meditation was proven to be an effective way of reducing stress and helping to boost the immune system thus helping to reduce pain and more effectively fight disease. The opponents of meditation who had stated that “meditation was not proven to be effective” were silenced by this research. This should have been a wake up call for governments trying to reduce the escalating costs of healthcare. Unfortunately the official reaction to this medical breakthrough has been slow to glacial.

How many other non-patentable products and services could be proven to be effective if research was undertaken? In my estimation, there are many.

Having read a considerable volume of supposedly "non-reputable" research my conclusion is that healthcare has taken a wrong turn. This is because governments have abdicated their responsibility for developing and funding a research strategy. Health care research has had to rely on obtaining funds from corporations that benefit from patents. Corporations that have in the past warped the ethics of research are now in control of healthcare research.

We are paying the price for this abdicated strategy, healthcare has become difficult to afford and the high cost is destroying socialized medicine. Just look at the increases in costs in healthcare in the last few decades, and look at the proportional distribution of that increase related to the rising costs of prescription drugs . Drug costs in Canada were rising so fast hospitals were facing, double digit annual inflation for drugs, while receiving budget increases around 2%. This disparity between costs and system funding resulted in the health system downloading much of these costs to individual consumers. Apparently patients die because they cannot afford the drugs. The CMAJ study in 2012 showed that 10% of Canadians could not afford prescription drugs. The same story is being repeated around the world.

To conclude, what does all this mean to you in doing your due diligence research into cancer treatment? It means:

- Look for results in both reputable and more obscure journals.
- Is there replicability? (i.e. in more than one article).

- Follow the money trail (who benefits from the product or who's ox is gored by the research?).
- Is the researcher well known? (follow the link on pubmed for their name).
- Was the research done by a reputable organization, university or government agency?
- Lastly, does it sound good? By this we mean, what is your gut reaction to this? We often hear of interesting findings, but many of them are "tomato" findings (everyone who eats a tomato will die!). Everyone who goes into remission may have had a cold at some point, but it doesn't mean that having colds cured them. There again, it might!

It is very important for us to stress how important this component of your research is. Doing your due diligence is a key component in your strategy to beat the odds. Be creative with your searches, look up those crazy ideas on the internet and check out the research. Now you understand how to use Pubmed, by all means use any search engine to get ideas, then check them out on Pubmed or a similar scholarly research site. Research everything, what you eat, supplements that might help, how to reduce stress, how to stay positive, alternative and "complementary" treatments, side effects, as well as the treatments your doctor is recommending.

Being both optimistic and skeptical is healthy. So keep following the research.

Free Updating Service

Another very useful tool we use regularly is the internet alert systems. Google alerts for example will send you free daily or weekly news updates for any topic you want. For example you can get google to send you information on; breast cancer, cancer genetics, foods that fight cancer, etc.. We constantly use many of these free updates to keep current with medical findings that have been reported in the news. We double check the results on Pubmed and other scientific services.

The alerts are delivered to your email account as frequently as you want, daily may be too frequent, weekly works well. These alerts are free, and you can have as many as you want. You can modify, add or delete searches regularly.

The results are presented in the form of links. When you click on these you get more information that is mainly taken from internet and published media sources. Using these alerts, you won't miss a suspected breakthrough or potential opportunity to do something that may help you beat the odds.

One that arrived as the book was being edited (February 13, 2012) was an interesting article about some Israeli researchers who have developed a blood test to detect cancer before symptoms appear. This research is worth following over the next few years since if successful it could lead to early intervention. The earlier you start using the techniques in this book the more likely you will be to prevent cancer or slow cancer cell growth so follow their work.

Another important aid to understanding the research is to use a good online health care dictionary, check out the National Library of Medicine sites such as “Med-line Plus”. Every time my family health team advises me to have a blood test, we ask them for a copy of the results then look up what the results mean online, the National Library of medicine site is excellent. So, for example, what is a lymphocyte? What does it mean when your RBC (red blood count) is low? Don’t be put off by the use of words you don’t understand, empower yourself through knowledge that is free. Create your own glossary of terms you frequently come across if that is helpful.

Put together a binder to keep your notes, your questions, your feelings together and take that with you to your medical appointments. Read it occasionally to track your progress. Having a well documented source of issues you are facing will also ensure you don’t forget to discuss all issues with your healthcare team.

In conclusion, take the time to do your research extensively, make lists of your questions, don’t accept vague answers and if you feel something isn’t right do more research and/or get a second opinion.

The links mentioned in this chapter are included in the resource section in appendix two.

CHAPTER TWO - Strategy

"Strategy without tactics is
the slowest route to victory.
Tactics without strategy is
the noise before defeat."
Sun Tzu

Your cancer strategy is your plan to achieve your long term goal, a return to health; your tactics are the individual actions you will take to get there. You need an overall plan and you need to put it in writing. Taking action without a plan is not going to help you achieve your goal as easily.

You have been diagnosed with cancer. You need a plan to help you move forward. The alternative is to put yourself completely in someone else's hands. This option is not great unless that person is extremely competent, is available 24 hours a day, seven days a week and always has your best interests at heart. You are the best person to lead that role, so how do you proceed?

Initially you need time to take stock. Ask yourself if you are having an emotional reaction. It is natural to have one. Give yourself permission to be fearful, or astonished or angry. Read chapter eight and heed the suggestion that if you are finding this overwhelming you may need to reach out for help.

Chapter one will have helped you to gain the knowledge and perspective you need to understand your situation. Keep reading relevant articles in medical journal articles and set up google alerts so that you are notified if new information about your form of cancer is making the news.

It is important for you to understand what your health team knows. You may initially find what they have to say confusing, so the more informed you are the better you will understand what they are saying. Take notes or record your sessions with your medical team or take along a friend who can take notes for you so you will be able to analyze or review everything they have said later.

Key Questions To Help Create Your Strategy

Ask yourself these key questions:

- **Are you sure that your diagnosis is a fact or do you need a second opinion?** Some diagnoses are difficult to make. A good clinician will have informed you of any doubts. For example, a high reading for a blood or urine analysis will need a second test since such tests are notorious for false readings. Biopsies are tests on your tissue and are usually much more reliable. Ask questions.
- **Are you knowledgeable enough?** Once we become convinced that our diagnosis is true, we now need to completely understand that diagnosis. Start information gathering. Ignore any predictions of death, we are interested in beating the odds, not believing statistics that

are notoriously bad. Chapter one will have taught you how to find scientific information upon which you will build your knowledge base.

- **Are you positive?** You have just been slapped in the face by the reality of a diagnosis and our first task is to stay positive. Chapter eight has been written to help you understand and deal with stress. In this regard, for now, stay away from negative people. Stressed individuals will bring you down, as will those who are flippant. One person on hearing I had cancer said to my face, oh that doesn't surprise me you are so overweight. Another said, oh, maybe you have done all you came here to do, another that it was bad karma from a past life. Just stay away from people like this for now. Later, once you have built up your strength you will be able to deal with them or laugh it all off.
- **Are your information sources solid?** You need to make sure your information sources are not biased, ill informed or have an agenda. Remember what you learned in chapter one and find out how your information sources are funded. Use the information sources listed in Appendix Two our Resources Section.
- **Do you have a good team of people to help you fight this fight?** Even if you have a medical degree you need a team of people to get you through this. Read chapter three for suggestions on how to build your team. It is key to take someone with you to see your oncologist/ specialist. No matter how tough you are, this can be an emotional roller coaster and you need someone who is level headed to

listen to the specialists, make notes and ask questions that you may be temporarily unable to ask. We would also strongly recommend purchasing a portable recorder so you can play back your physician patient conversations. All too often the stress associated with these interactions makes your recall less than perfect.

- **Does your current diet fight cancer or feed it?** You don't have to become vegan or go on a weird diet to embrace a cancer fighting diet. In most cases you simply need to cut some foods out and add some cancer fighting foods. Chapter four is about cancer fighting foods and why these are important as part of your cancer therapy. You are what you eat, so create an environment in your body that cancer finds difficult to thrive in, don't give cancer an easy ride.
- **How is your mental toughness?** This is a defining moment in your life. Everything you have ever done or believed will come to mind. Don't give up. How can you improve your mental stability and strength, chapter eight is written to help you with this. Suspend your disbelief, you may benefit from considering options you haven't considered in your life so far.
- Ensure your **family members are OK?** Tell your family members to go for a check up and get screened for cancer. Tell your sons and daughters so they are screened on a regular basis by their family physicians. .***"Many more patients would survive cancer if doctors screened those families at highest risk."*** This recent quote was from researchers who found that in certain types of cancer

heredity was often a significant component. So if you are a family member of someone with cancer, clearly one of your strategies should be to arrange to be screened more often than other people.

- **Is your team looking after you?** The health system doesn't act like a fully integrated health organization should. In an ideal world everyone in your health team would be fully informed, they would read your chart, communicate with each other and create a unique path and strategy for your return to full health. Well, unless you are very rich and can afford to hire the best health professionals privately this is unlikely to happen. Even if you have lots of money, like Michael Jackson, you may fall prey to doctors with ethical challenges. So read chapter three carefully, you need to develop a plan that is unique for you. Until all healthcare professionals have access to your health record you will need to ensure your team members receive all clinical information that is relevant for your care so they can work with you to achieve your goals.
- **Are you keenly aware of what is going on?** You may become easily confused due to chemotherapy or for other reasons. Do you have a health advocate or health system navigator who can help you when you are not at your best? Health professionals are human, they make mistakes. No matter how good their intentions may be, the systems and the people in it are not perfect, follow-up is not always done swiftly and cutbacks can eliminate benefits that used

to exist. The bottom line is that the system may drop the ball so;

We need to take responsibility for our own care.

This statement means that our own personal unique team needs to take that responsibility. If you assume that the system will take care of you, you are risking your health and your opportunity to "beat the odds".

- **Is your expert, expert enough?** Each health discipline has a body of knowledge on which their expertise is based. Unless you are dealing with an exceptional health professional they most likely will not be highly knowledgeable of the latest information in other disciplines.

If you are in doubt, get a referral to another expert and/or get a second opinion.

Sometimes you will need another kind of expert. A friend of mine researches cancer care for patients with multiple illnesses. So, if you have diabetes and heart disease and then get cancer you will need an expert like him to sort out what works and what doesn't. If you have multiple issues, you should probably ask to be seen by an expert at an academic health sciences centre since your family doctor is unlikely to have the expertise or time to expertly manage your care path through the group of experts you may require.

- **Do your experts have the right attitude?**

Some (others may say most) health professionals are arrogant. They are taught that they are the cream that rose to the top. Some are right! There are some very bright individuals who are health professionals! This doesn't give them the right to be arrogant, but some of them think that it does. They get away with it since they are good clinicians. In small communities they get away with it since it is sometimes more difficult to recruit doctors and people are willing to settle for what they have. Several individuals we interviewed told us hair raising stories of arrogance and tolerated incompetence.

This arrogance creates situations where the physicians believe their own press! In other words they begin to think they always have the right answer and anything you or another health professional comes up with is wrong. This is both dangerous to your health and frustrating to deal with. Deal with it you must, either find a way of opening the discussion or change health professionals.

They are also taught that how you say something is as important as what you say. The result is that it is in your best interests not to react, but to check out what they recommend. In other words;

- ***Are you verifying information?.***

This is very difficult for some people to grasp. People especially from older generations were taught to respect people with education and position. This is quite appropriate, unless they are wrong! If they are commenting outside their field of expertise the likelihood of them being wrong increases.

People have died by listening to bad advice that they were too shy to question. This situation can be difficult when you live in a small town with few doctors and you don't want them to treat you badly because you questioned their opinion. You have to make a choice, sometimes you need to go to a larger centre. A move to a city is sometimes healthier than staying put. Fortunately most health professionals go into their careers for the right reasons and you won't need to do this.

Anne was concerned about her mother who had fallen several times. Another healthcare team member found a medication error. Anne was afraid to tell the prescribing physician they had made a mistake because she feared "bad feelings" might result in her mother receiving less than stellar care. She confided that the belief in this small town was that you need to be careful you didn't annoy the doctors or you would find it difficult to get an appointment when you needed one.

- ***Are you taking this seriously enough?***

Everyone reacts differently to a diagnosis. One group just laughs it off. This is clearly a bad choice. They seem to feel this will go away just like the flu has gone away in the past.

A second group goes into denial (no, not the river in Egypt!). Some individuals do fail to hear the bad news from doctors, they don't tell their spouses and they don't take any corrective action. If I stick my head in the sand the cancer can't see me.

Both are good reasons to take a friend along to every specialist appointment.

Unfortunately, individuals in denial probably won't read this book but if your spouse or friend or close relative is in denial you may need to intervene. Chapter eight may help you if you must intervene.

- ***Do you have the resources you need?***

One of Paul's biggest surprises was that following the diagnosis he couldn't work yet his medical expenses soared. Even in a health system touted as providing universal coverage, his drugs weren't covered and they were expensive. Paul had to make significant life changes to afford to take the drugs.

It is not just drugs that may be excluded from your health coverage. Certain team members are also not covered by insurance or the health care system. Make sure you contact those who know about health professionals who offer pro-bono services or agencies that subsidize drugs, or drug companies that offer drug subsidies. Some drug companies are generous and do offer free drugs to those in need. Don't be shy about asking for help from agencies like the cancer society, they exist to help people like you and if they cannot help they usually know people or groups who can.

Nobody should die due to a lack of financial resources to buy treatment services or drugs, unfortunately one side effect of the expensive drug focussed culture is that many do.

- **Are we having fun yet?**

This is serious business so remember to stop and smell the roses, learn to laugh again, develop true happiness. Read chapter eight, visualize yourself being well again. In 2010 researchers finally confirmed what many had suspected, psychological stress is a potential trigger for cancer and stress will generate many chemicals which do not help fight cancer. Adrenaline for example accelerates tumor growth. Dealing with stress is both possible and achievable without drugs. You need to start now. Prevention is always better than the cure. Learning how to reduce stress and learning to laugh again can help you fight the spread and growth of cancer.

- **Are you full of hope?**

You will meet many types of people in a healthcare setting. The easy categorization from specialists we talked to and interviewed was ***that those with hope and a positive attitude live longer***. Most health professionals agree with this. Read chapter nine for more hope inspiring information.

Are you documenting it?

Start your journal and document your appointments, what was said, what your friend who went along with you heard, what your prescriptions are, what is your reaction to them. You will find that your team members do not remember everything and having a journal to refer to is useful for all.

Write how you feel, how your emotions are changing, the steps you are taking to review your emotions. Document research sites you have visited, bookmark good sites on your web browser. Write a newsletter like my friend Allan to tell your friends how you are doing (see appendix three). Let those emotions out, and you will find many friends who will support your efforts. A cancer diagnosis brings out the best in people, you will find support from places you never thought possible.

Your plan will change as your cancer progresses. There will be good days and not so good days. Have your tactics in place for the not so good days, who you will turn to and what you will do to remain positive and healthy.

Strategy in place? Now on to the actions to bring that strategy into being.

CHAPTER THREE - Building Your Team

"The good physician treats the disease; the great physician treats the patient who has the disease."
Sir William Osler

John told me that his physician was wonderful he was so good because he didn't tell, he asked. When John told his physician he was worried, the doc asked why, he didn't tell John not to worry, or give him false hope nor was he bluntly honest. John told me that his physician came across as his friend, not an arrogant bureaucrat or expert hiding behind his use of medical language.

Cancer cuts across many fields of study. No one person is an expert in "cancer", the subject is too broad for any person to understand everything. This is why we need a team of health professionals to care for us. Let us explore why this is important, and why you need to think outside the box in putting together your dream team to ensure you beat the odds.

First we will look at the system reasons for building a team so we understand why it is important.

Many years ago as part of his job the author had the opportunity to visit some US healthcare sites to observe health care delivery in some of the worlds premiere healthcare settings. The author visited the Mayo Clinic, Cleveland Clinic, Texas Heart Institute and Johns Hopkins Hospital on behalf of a Canadian teaching hospital.

By spending two or three days at each setting the author was able to follow patients throughout their diagnosis, clinic visits, lab tests, diagnostic testing and surgical stays. Patient flow through these systems was observed. The purpose was to see if there was anything we could learn from these world class organizations that could be implemented in Canada to improve the system for the benefit of patients.

The technology and speed of service at these places was unbelievable to a Canadian, originally from the UK, who regularly saw patients waiting weeks or months from initially seeing the family doctor to eventual treatment.

Patients were seen very quickly in most of these centres. At the Mayo Clinic for example, patients were seen one day and could be in the operating room the next day. Diagnostic tests were ordered and completed within 24 hours. The health centre even had a hotel with on call nurses for families and patient recovery in real comfort. On the surface it was a dream system, certainly a “Cadillac” of systems.

To achieve this speedy result the Clinic had to have a huge excess medical equipment capacity. One example, was that there were six times the number of Magnetic Resonance Imaging Machines (MRIs) than at a similar sized Canadian hospital. At the time (MRI'S) cost over $2 million a piece and over $100,000 a year to operate. Few places could afford such excess capacity. The Mayo Clinic was very well funded by well heeled corporations and donors who wanted and were prepared to pay for the very best service, with no waiting period.

These top end health care settings are luxurious compared to the charity clinics in many parts of the US. This was a system built for the rich and famous not for the "not for profit" Canadian system. Since the system I represented couldn't afford excess capacity, most of the ideas brought back were system related, not recommendations to build excess capacity.

In the social universal healthcare systems such as that in Canada the mortality and morbidity rates are similar to the US or in some cases actually better. Costs in the Canadian system are constrained by carefully managing the available resources. The average cost per patient is much less than the US and is more affordable as a national system.

Instead of excess capacity, Canada and the UK for example prioritize the patients by urgency. In this way urgent cases are seen first, often immediately or at least within days of identifying their need for testing and not so urgent cases wait. Other countries with universal health systems are very similar to the Canadian system using rationing and urgency ratings to ensure that patients don't become worse or die on a waiting list. Public pressure on the politicians ensures that new resources are added if the waiting lists become too long.

The point of this discussion is that in countries with socialized medicine the timelines can be longer. This is not a problem if you are waiting for non life threatening surgery (such as a knee replacement) but it can be an issue for some diagnoses.

Cancer crosses over many disciplines, this sometimes means that you may need to stay alert to prevent falling through the cracks. Here are some potential issues to keep in mind.

First, have you been told, or do you know whether a time delay will affect your outcome? This question is key, some cancers are quick growing, others slower, find out about yours. Obviously time is of the essence for all cancer but especially for faster growing cancers. If the actions of your medical team seems to be glacial,make sure your medical team knows you want faster treatment. As mentioned previously, ensure you have your medical record with you when you talk with other health professionals, waiting for records to be transferred can cause unnecessary delays in treatment.

One serious side effect of a managed system is that patients occasionally fall through the cracks. This will be cured by better computer tracking systems over time but for now, we often need to be the squeaky wheel to ensure we get the service we need in a timely manner. Take ownership, ask;

"what response time does the research indicate is needed?"

Also, watch the assumptions that are being made that may affect you. Some family doctors, for example, assume (or learned when last at school) that certain cancers are slow growing. This assumption has affected many people who actually had fast growing versions. For example, there are reportedly 25 types of prostate cancer alone. Some are fast growing, most are not. Your family practitioner may not have come across your faster growing variety before. Family practitioners have hundreds of patients with a wide variety of diseases, they cannot stay on top of all the research for all those diseases all the time. This is not a criticism but a side effect of the explosion in health information.

Remember you are the architect of your chances to beat the odds. Do you have the money to go elsewhere or can you raise the money if the system you are in is acting too slowly? Alternatively, can you make the system take notice and move faster? Can you ensure that you are being referred appropriately and in a timely fashion? Can you get help to assist you in moving the system along when it needs to move? Do not assume that the system will operate efficiently, most of the time it will, but take action if it does not.

" Scott, a psychologist reported the following. Paul contacted me, I had been helping him through some dark times.

"My family doctor sent me for an ultrasound, do I have cancer?"

"What did your doctor say?"

"He didn't say anything."

"Did you ask him anything?"

"No, he just told me I needed an ultrasound."

"Did he do a DRE?"

"Whats that?"

"Did he do a digital rectal exam?"

"Whats that?"

"Did he stick his finger where the sun don't shine?"

"Yes"

"Did he say anything?"

"No, he just told me to go for an ultrasound"

"What did the ultrasound order form say?"

"Couldn't read it, but my wife thought it said enlarged, does that mean I have cancer?"

"No, could just be BPH, benign prostatic hyperplasia, there are medications and supplements that can help that. Did he order a PSA?"

"What's that?"

"So it went, according to Paul, the doctor had explained little, Paul was very scared. It was triggering his previous bout of depression. Whether this was Paul's imaginings or a doctor who communicates badly is unknown!"

This story illustrates the importance of having a friend with you at key healthcare meetings.

It is as true in health care as in most areas of life, that the squeaky wheel gets the oil. Are you therefore pushing to get information, to be seen, diagnosed, treated? Are you politely demanding an explanation you can understand for the course of treatment being prescribed?

Some health professionals have biases towards young vibrant, good looking, charismatic patients (this is well documented in the literature) so if you are not in this category for some reason you may need to push harder to get equal access. This may be the role for your **advocate or health system navigator**. This is a very key position, in my case filled by my beautiful wife Elizabeth who was both a nurse and health administrator. You definitely would benefit from having someone like her on your team.

Initially, my oncologist was very excited to include me in a clinical trial and I had lots of attention from assistants until it was discovered that my cancer had metastasized. The attention then disappeared overnight.

My case no longer fit the criteria for the study. So in addition to having to deal with a cancer that was more serious than expected, I also found myself struggling to figure out why I couldn't get answers from the health care assistants anymore. In addition, I was left figuring out why the former excitement had evaporated.

If you have the opportunity to be part of a clinical trial, give that serious consideration, you will be tracked and served well. So, to beat the odds try to find a clinical trial for your type of cancer and try to get the physician running it to see if you can be included. If you are excluded for some reason, be the squeaky wheel and ensure you still get good treatment anyway.

Your health team needs to be involved with you on this journey, it is not enough for them to just do their job. Cancer symptoms often include fatigue, depression and memory issues, so you need people to support you and take up the slack. In Nova Scotia, Canada for example they have nurse navigators to help people navigate through the system. This is a great way to ensure timely coordination and gives the patient someone to rely on. You may know health professionals who are willing to volunteer their help. Sometimes all you have to do is ask. Look to volunteer associations, especially the local cancer societies, churches, and other charitable organizations. Don't be shy about asking, there are thousands of wonderful people out there willing to help you, just remember to treat them with the respect they deserve.

Cancer "Deafness"

One story I heard from many of my Oncologist friends was that they really do try to be very sensitive when giving patients bad news. They take time in a quiet environment, they explain all of the possible options and outcomes and they try to give hope when it is reasonable to do so. However, they report that when the family doctor next meets with the patient and asks what the Oncologist said the usual response is "he told me I have cancer", did he say anything else? "Not that I remember".

What has happened in these situations is that the trauma of learning the bad news is so stressful that it literally blocks out all other memories from that encounter. This is a well documented phenomenon. The trauma of being told you have cancer can be similar to being in a car accident in terms of the acute stress load and memory loss.

So next time you hear that an Oncologist wasn't communicative, check it out for yourself. Doctors are often unfairly labelled as having poor bedside manners when the reality is that almost anyone giving bad news will be perceived as being cold. We also need to realize that this is not the fun part of their job, and that some do it better than others. Remember, poor bedside manners does not necessarily mean they are bad doctors, some of the best surgeons for example are poor communicators.

Clearly this is very important; take a friend with you to these key meetings. We don't hear well when we are stressed, afraid, or when we are hearing technical terms. Take someone who will not be too emotional, preferably someone who has health care experience, can understand medical jargon and who can take notes. Take a tape recorder and record your medical visit if you cannot take along a friend.

Which Doctor (Not Witch Doctor)

Which brings me to that old healthcare joke...

There are over 2,000 medical schools world wide that graduate doctors annually.

Question; What do you call the person who graduated bottom of their class at the worst medical school in the world?

Answer; Doctor.

So the point is that there are extreme situations where you may get a poorly prepared doctor and you may need a second opinion. This can be difficult. Here is Peter's example;

"After having a bad experience with one doctor I asked another organization for a second opinion. My insurer, wanted my family doctor to make the referral, so I then found myself back to a family doctor to explain the situation. Fortunately my family health team is helpful and that was no problem, but we have heard that some family practitioners take being gate keepers very seriously and like to exert the little authority they have and can make life difficult for their patients. In my case, the second opinion was worth having, the second team made several suggestions that positively crossed the line of the ordinary and treatment was pursued. What if I had accepted the first opinion and done nothing? I am told I would be dead today. In this case the second opinion not only worked but I believe it went a long way towards helping me to extend my life!"

My advice is to stand up for yourself, and get your friends to help you make your argument if that is necessary. In most private and social healthcare systems you have the right to ask for a second opinion, use it when necessary but don't abuse it

The next point is what to do if you suspect you should be being seen, and due to circumstances cannot be seen or cannot get a referral. There are organizations that can help. Don't be afraid or too proud to ask for help. Try your local cancer societies, church, seniors centre, member of parliament, see if the system you are in has "ombudspersons", contact your local hospital. Become the squeaky wheel, make these organizations part of your team.

Having friends in the health system can be a blessing or a curse depending on who they are, where they work and how much influence they have. You don't want to annoy the people who are trying to help you. In addition you do not want to become labeled as a whiner or complainer. That being said, this is your life. It is worth fighting for and if you come across a negative attitude, ask them;

"What would you do if you were in my situation?"

This often results in double takes, but it usually helps. They take their answers a little more seriously when you bring their life into the equation. Remember, in the preparation of bacon and eggs for breakfast, the hen is involved, the pig is committed. The health professionals are the hens and you are the pig. The hens see so many people that they sometimes forget what it is like to be the pig and to have your life on the line. Fortunately however most health professionals are compassionate and caring.

So, now you are empowered to take on difficult health professionals if you need to, who else should you have on your "dream team"?

Dream Team

So here are a few suggestions for your dream team to support you with your cancer diagnosis and treatment.

First, your friends and relatives can be a good source of help. Six degrees of separation will bring you to other people with cancer diagnoses, people who work in healthcare and others who can give wise counsel. My wife is from a healthcare background, as am I so we know lots of people who gave great advice and we are very thankful. So reach out for help, as soon as people find you need help wonderful people come out of the woodwork. Ask them to help, this is not the time to be bashful (or any of the other 7 dwarfs for that matter!).

My personal Angel and dream team leader is my spouse Elizabeth. This is her story.

"A cancer diagnosis has a devastating effect on the individual diagnosed with cancer and their entire family including their spouse. Often times the ill spouse cannot work, in addition some cancer drug treatments are not funded by the healthcare system. These

types of issues are common experiences and put a financial and emotional burden on both the patient and the spouse. This is the stressful environment that a family can find themselves in when a cancer diagnosis strikes. A cancer diagnosis can threaten your entire way of life. Often the diagnosis requires the family to evaluate everything that they once took for granted and make some significant life adjustments.

As Michael's spouse I was devastated to learn of his cancer. We had worked flat out our entire lives running a health consulting and software development company and raising three children. We had always dreamt of our retirement together and now we were forced to consider a much shorter life for Michael and me growing old alone. It was devastating to consider life without my partner and soul mate. This realization strengthened my resolve as the spouse of a cancer patient to do everything in my power to help my husband beat the odds.

When we received the cancer diagnosis the first thing Michael and I did was educate ourselves so that we could actively beat the death sentence. We purchased books on foods that fight cancer and searched the internet to strengthen our knowledge so we could discover strategies that might help us beat the odds.

The literature was very clear, a large proportion of cancers and chronic disease in our society are lifestyle related. Working at a desk, on flights and in meetings, 10 to 12 hours a day and ignoring diet and exercise was killing my husband. This realization made it clear that lifestyle adjustments needed to be made and I could really help my husband by participating in these fully, exercising together daily and changing our diet so that it consisted mainly of foods that fight cancer.

At the beginning of Michael's cancer therapy I was upset because I could not take every day off work and take my husband to radiation therapy. I needed to continue to work and earn money to support our family. Thanks to our wonderful church community many friends volunteered to support us and took Michael to and from his radiation appointments. With that incredible support network in place I was able *to continue working and use my time to make serious changes in our diet. The other way that I felt part of my husbands cancer journey was by giving him daily Reiki to ease the discomfort of his daily radiation therapy. It was empowering to be able to ease his pain through Reiki healing and to make him stronger by changing our diet so it included foods that truly fight cancer.*

As an active participant in Michael's strategy to beat the odds I felt like we had some control over the outcome of his therapy and as a former nurse I needed to participate in my husband's cancer journey."

You may need to change the way you approach health issues, I know my original reaction was to decline help since I had always been on the other side of this fence. Accepting help was hard initially until someone pointed out I was being too proud for my own good. Point taken, I started accepting the help, offers to drive me to my radiation sessions poured in, offers of food and companionship. My wife pointed out to me that people wanted to help, it wasn't an imposition, it actually helped them too! Healthcare friends suggested people I could call and sources of information. It felt good once I learned to accept assistance. Sometimes in life we have to accept that we cannot do it alone. If you have been diagnosed with cancer and need help, now is one of those times. Enlist your friends to help you change.

Cancer is triggered by a variety of things including stress, heredity or toxins (see appendix one for more information on cancer triggers). If you were dealt a poor hand in the heredity department or are a victim of workplace exposure to toxins you may benefit from the help of others who have gone through a similar situation and may have solutions you haven't thought of.

Naturopaths

Ian tells us;I took the advice and checked out the naturopathic college. My initial reaction was not to contact the naturopathic college, a relative had had a very bad experience.

My attitude, as the license plates from the state of Missouri say, was "show me". Fortunately they took me at my word, the student I was assigned at the naturopathic college took me very literally and every time we met provided me with pages of references for every supplement and recommendation she made. I took each of these sheets home and immediately went on the medical search engines (mentioned in chapter one) *and looked them up to see what the evidence based research was saying.*

As they say in the UK, I was "gob smacked". The papers they referred to were on the whole, very reputable, many were from main stream medical journals that were peer reviewed. Some were from lesser known universities, most were replicated by other researchers. Although understandably not "double blind" none of the references were "flaky". This was the opposite of what I had expected."

Clearly there is some excellent research in the naturopathic area that isn't being communicated to patients who stay solely within the "medical" system.

Sometimes it takes being ill yourself to realize what works best. Like Ian,having this realization myself was a major incentive to write this book. Patients would benefit and many more would "beat the odds" if naturopaths and other health professionals worked more closely together.

The good news for all of us is that there are many aspects of a naturopathic practitioners care that can be very helpful to you in beating the odds. My recommendation is that you follow the "I'm from Missouri" approach, get the naturopath to show you the proof, and be healthily skeptical as Ian was. Check out the references before you commit to the supplements and practices they recommend.

Dietary Advice

Diet has been determined to be one of the most important determinants of health.

When I read "Foods that Fight Cancer" by Beliveau and Gingras I realized two things. First, my wife and mother had been right, I had been eating all wrong for most of my life, and second, there is a scientific basis to much of what dietitians, nutritionists and others had been recommending. I needed to change my diet.

You probably need to change yours.

Apparently you are what you eat, and consequently I was sandwiches, beef and french fries washed down with beer, with none of that rabbit food if you please. It was no wonder I was overweight and unhealthy.

George realized that he needed a food expert on his team ASAP. You probably need one too.

"From a food perspective I was as complete an idiot as you can find. This change was not easy."

The best advice comes from dietitians, nutritional counsellors and nutritionists. My hospital didn't offer one, although I found out later that I could have consulted one if I had asked. Another lesson in taking charge of your own future. Many exist in private practice, or in organizations like Wellspring or the Haven which are organizations specifically created to support cancer patients and their families (links for these resources are found in Appendix two). My naturopath was a great source of dietary recommendations. So between her, my own research and my wife and mother, I had dietary support on my team. It was quite the learning experience!

Exercise Coach

Exercise sucks, my first negative exposure to exercise began in high school in the UK when gym and field exercise was mandatory. The teacher was a monster who enjoyed torturing little boys with rope climbing, rugby, throwing the shot and most boring of all cricket. The only time I did well was throwing the javelin; he walked along the perimeter of the pitch and was laughing at our efforts, I missed him by inches. I amazed myself and him! Perhaps understandably, our relationship went further downhill from there.

Later in life, my children embarrassed me into doing karate and that was good exercise for a few years. Other than karate and Tai Chi I had successfully avoided exercise for many years, and my pant waist size attested to that. It seemed to grow an inch each year along with my age!

The research is clear, fat people are more likely to get cancer. That moron who rudely told me just after I was diagnosed that I had contracted cancer because I was fat was factually correct, even if they could benefit from some lessons in diplomacy.

So exercise is clearly something we need to understand. A personal trainer helps, add them to your team if you can afford one. If not get a friend who likes to walk, to drop by your house every day and take you walking. My dog does that for me, he whines at me until I take him out. So I added my dog to my team.

Other Team Members

" In the last week, we have met the occupational therapist who is now part of our care team, and today, we will have our first visit with our personal support worker, who will be coming in twice a week to give me some time to focus on other things that

need doing. Last night, my husband slept through the night for the first time in a very long time!"

Home care is another great source of help, you may benefit from them being on your team if you qualify. Give them as much lead time as you can since it can take time to be approved for this support.

If you are anything other than completely happy, you need to see a psychologist. Cancer is said to cause depression, it may also be true that depression triggers cancer. Either way, if you are in the slightest unhappy, see a psychologist or psychiatrist. Cancer has ways of bringing up issues you have avoided, like the eventuality of your death and your future without a job to name two. Continuing to avoid these issues may contribute to unhappiness. By the way, read my last book; "Meditation for Enduring Happiness" for hints to keep you very happy.

Who else do you need? The medical specialists come with the diagnosis. Get to know them, study what they are supposed to know. Challenge them with questions, make yourself an interesting patient by asking questions that show you are engaged, you will get a better response.

You may need a social worker. Social workers focus on improving your quality of life by helping you solve problems such as where to find funding, transportation, how to get home based care, how to get into long term care,. . .

Free volunteer help abounds, some organizations offer free courses in meditation, diet counseling, financial assistance, etc. They are more abundant in large cities. One called Wellspring in Canada is a great cancer support agency. Haven in the UK is a great breast Cancer support agency. The resource section Appendix Two provides links to these and other resources. Ask around, your full time job right now is getting well, so investigate every resource you can.

Churches can be very helpful, my wife and I have sung in church choir for many years. Church communities can be very supportive. The last church we attended had a parish nurse for a while. Parish nurses are often fully qualified nurses who will help anyone in the parish who needs assistance. They can be a great resource helping individuals to navigate the system.

There are numerous community agencies who would like to help you, get a list from the local cancer agencies and local government. While often short on funds, the individuals in these agencies are usually great people who have learned how to creatively mold the system to meet peoples needs, it is worth your while to meet them.

Other helpers may come from a variety of sources; Yoga groups, service clubs, other volunteer agencies. My church community lined up a long list of volunteers to drive me to radiation and there were so many volunteers I had a hard time arranging a ride with each one over the thirty nine days of radiation. May you be so lucky, not only did these volunteers get me to my necessary appointments, they provided emotional support during the most vulnerable period of my treatment, when I was anemic, weak and very tired. Their contribution to my mental health was invaluable. Thank you all.

CHAPTER FOUR - Food As Medicine

Food can be powerful medicine, basic nutrition or a form of cancer promoting poison, your choice.

"Having just read" Foods that Fight Cancer" we discussed the book and he purchased it. The next week he was feeling much better. He had consumed less junk food, more fruit, veggies, nuts and whole grains and he had more energy. Why hadn't the health system told him this when he was diagnosed he asked? Good question."

My parents are alive and well and in their mid eighties. There is no history of prostate cancer in my family as far back as four generations, beyond that we don't have the information. Yet I was diagnosed with metastatic prostate cancer at age 58 and my youngest sister lost her battle with breast cancer and died at age 47. In both our cases environmental toxins are the most likely trigger and experts say they probably came in food.

This is the point where a medical expert might interject. She/he would be correct in saying that the human body is amazing in that it has a built in filter system for toxins. They refer to the liver and kidneys, organs that filter the blood and remove toxins in a normal patient.

"Ay, there's the rub" as the opening soliloquy of Act 3 Scene 1 Hamlet says, it would seem that our modern world is filled with abnormal livers and kidneys. The proliferation of chemicals and saturated fat in the diet of the modern world seems to have confounded the normal liver and kidneys. It has recently been determined for example, that diabetes can cause non alcoholic fatty liver disease. The estimated 285 million people worldwide with diabetes may have abnormal livers, and that is not to mention all the alcoholic livers and kidneys.

The prevalence of fatty liver disease in the western world varies from 30-60% of the population, depending on the study you read. A recent study in non-developed countries found levels generally below 10% but rising. The point is we are dealing with a whole new world when it comes to "medical normal". Diseased livers and kidneys don't filter toxins as effectively as healthy ones. It is therefore no surprise that individuals with chronic diseases such as diabetes have a higher chance of getting cancer.

A Japanese man living in Japan has one eightieth the chance of contracting prostate cancer as the North American man according to the Cancer Society, yet if he moves to North America he has the same chance as a North American man. So is it our lifestyle, our food, our environment, or something we haven't thought of? We don't know for sure but a prime suspect is food, because prepared and fast foods contain chemical preservatives that some consider toxins, saturated fats and excessive amounts of sugars or sugar substitutes.

Our North American diet is about 30-40% fat, other countries with lower cancer rates run about 20% fat. Of course it is not just fat but also the type of fat. My family is from a fishing town in England. We ate fish several times a week and ate the more expensive red meat once or twice a week. This may explain why our family was perfectly healthy until we came to North America. Experts tell us that fish oils are good oils, while red meat and dairy fats are bad fats. Fish is expensive in our part of North America and red meat is relatively inexpensive, hence our family began eating more red meat in North America. We barbecued for the first time when we arrived in Canada. Charred red meat is more of a carcinogen too.

Red meat and fat is just the tip of the iceberg. North Americans and many Europeans are obese and often eat "comfort food" over good food. We are bombarded by 50 to 3,000 ads per day, depending on what we do and where we live, many of these ads are about fast food, usually the kind of food that is not good for us.

Tibetan monks are taught to think of food as medicine. If it doesn't serve a good purpose don't eat it. That takes will power, if like me you were told you were palliative, you have the incentive born of medical trauma to very quickly switch to healthy food. My recommendation is that if we were a lot more like those tibetan monks and chose to ignore the commercials for fast food we would all be a lot healthier. Food really is medicine, bad or good.

You are what you eat, and for most North Americans that means we are fat, greasy, toxic and consume too much sugar.

Again, my wonderful spouse Elizabeth:

"I had grown up in North America to a mother of Irish background. Meat and potatoes were staples of our diet and I had learned to cook the same way as my mother. Following Michael's diagnosis, clearly this was going to have to change because the literature was clear foods that fight cancer are mainly fruits, vegetables and spices. To get Michael to buy into these dietary changes I knew I would need to make vegetables taste great. Not only did they have to taste great I would need to balance carbohydrates with proteins to satisfy a big mans appetite and give him the necessary energy to fight the disease. I went on a quest to find excellent vegetarian cook books so I could create meals with foods that fight cancer. My favorite cook books are listed in Appendix Two the resource section of this book for your reference. Interesting to me is that since the diagnosis Michael and I have had the pleasure of going on Yoga Buddhist retreats and most of the great vegetarian food we have experienced have been on these retreats.

Survival is a strong instinct in all of us and Michael and I were in survival mode. We cut out red meat altogether, added more fish and made fruits and vegetables the mainstay of our diet. During the adjustment period Michael's naturopath asked him if he ever had tried to lose weight. Like many other North Americans Michael had tried numerous diets with few positive results. When the naturopath heard this she encouraged Michael to be tested for food sensitivities because consumption of foods you are even mildly allergic to can be a factor in obesity. Food sensitivity testing is unfortunately not a service covered by our Canadian healthcare system but it was a necessary test to make Michael more healthy and the testing revealed that he was allergic to more than 40 foods. Not only did we need to cut out red meat, we had to cut out most grain products like breads and cereal because of a gluten allergy.

We discovered that Michael was allergic to a range of fruits, vegetables and herbs. Fruits and vegetables like grapes, mangoes, tomatoes, mushrooms, carrots, peas, and garlic were on his allergy list and the list went on. I found this news devastating, for 30 years of married life I had been poisoning my spouse by feeding him things he was allergic to.

After Michael's allergies were identified we were asked to avoid all foods he was allergic to for six months. I became depressed because a huge range of vegetables that are the backbone of vegetarian cooking needed to be cut out. I challenge you try and find vegetarian stock that does not have carrots or tomatoes in the base. Try and find juice that does not include grape or blackberry juice. I read every label at the grocery store and modified the majority of new recipes I had uncovered so that there might be something we could eat. For many of you food allergies might not be an issue but if you have ever had problems losing weight, if you have noticed a burning sensation when you consume some foods or gastrointestinal upsets after eating certain foods you should seriously consider being allergy tested.

I never would have predicted what happened next. With the removal of foods Michael was allergic to he started to lose weight and for the first time in his life he didn't always feel ravenously hungry. The loss of weight gave him some more energy which I am convinced helped him through the fatigue of daily radiation therapy. I am not certain Michael would have been able to make these important dietary adjustments alone and it gave me a very positive way to contribute to my husband's cancer therapy.

Our diet changed from eggs and bacon or cereal and toast in the morning to fresh fruit and yogurt topped with nuts. Lunch went from being store bought soup and sandwiches to home made soups or a plate of fresh vegetables with healthy homemade dips like black bean dip and hummus. Dinners were often totally vegetarian like black bean gluten free pie and sweet potatoes or fish and vegetables. The quantity of vegetables in our diet grew exponentially and the spices used in cooking included turmeric and ginger *thanks to my new food bible "The Foods that Fight Cancer".*

The foods that I now cook are a far cry from those my mother made and I can honestly say that I don't think Michael or I miss red meat or packaged/ processed foods. Cooking takes longer but I know that what I am doing is making a real difference, I am helping my husband beat the odds."

Blobs R Us

Many people in developed countries think of food as a reward, comfort food. We eat because we are addicted to food; we eat to satisfy our emotional needs. Anyway the advertisements tell us to eat what makes us feel good.

The huge change we need to make after being diagnosed with cancer is to begin to think of food as medicine. So how do we eliminate the toxic food and start eating foods that fight cancer?

First, go to reliable sources, peer reviewed studies on Pubmed, Cancer society experts with an academic record, your health team who have had lessons in nutrition. Obtain books like "Foods that Fight Cancer".

Chemotherapy, is the taking of chemical preparations to fight cancer. What are cancer fighting foods? On a molecular level food is chemotherapy too. So if the food doesn't contradict your current therapy and it fights cancer it is just like that chemotherapy you need to receive, why aren't you taking it instead of eating junk? Considering our strategy for "beating the odds", after medical therapy, food as good medicine is the next most important thing.

So certain foods fight cancer by creating a positive environment that is not conducive to cancer cell proliferation, by actually killing cancer cells or by helping to cut off the blood supply cancer cells need. Green tea for example has been shown to kill cancer cells in the lab.

Cancer rates have increased threefold over the last fifty years. The only exceptions being those cancers caused by smoking, viral infections and a few others that have been helped by medical breakthroughs. The increase in the other cancers is thought to be attributable to toxins in the environment and food. Polluting corporations deny this, no surprise there. The tobacco industry denied any wrong doing for years and this strategy worked for them in the short term. Just as the citizens of Rome died from lead poisoning we are dying from corporate pollution. It is time for change.

What does this mean to those of us who are trying to beat the odds? It means we must source foods with lower toxicity levels. For example, Tuna has high mercury levels, so you should limit the quantity of Tuna you eat, eat other fish. Organic vegetables in areas where the organic growers are regulated have fewer toxins. Ask your local farmer what chemicals he/she uses and buy chemical free foods where possible. Wash your fruit and vegetables with soap and water or a vinegar and lemon solution to remove chemical residues. Lobby the government to better regulate the use of chemicals and additives in the food industry.

Water is natures way of flushing toxins from the body and helping the liver and kidneys do their job. Most of us don't drink enough water, we wait until we are thirsty, but often we are quite dehydrated before becoming thirsty. Symptoms of dehydration can be headaches, fatigue, joint or back pain and even dry skin. If you are constipated or your urine is darker than normal you may need to drink more. Talk to your team about what amount is right for you and make sure you drink enough water.

My personal process of changing to a cancer fighting yet tasty diet continues. The first six months were the worst, all my favourite foods were gone; chips, beer, wine, chocolate.

Your list may be quite different depending on your cancer type, allergies or sensitivities, and the severity of the cancer. Remember what I said about denial (not the river in Egypt), my suggestion is to ask for help from someone in your team who knows about your cancer and allergies, such as your nutrition therapist or naturopath.

Here are some basic guidelines to follow to create your own list.

1. Start gently by trying to eliminate "bad" stuff like trans fats, high cholesterol, very sweet or "rich" foods, white sugar.

2. Increase the proportion of vegetables in your daily intake. The evidence in favour of increasing certain fruits and vegetables to fight cancer is overwhelming. Science tells us

they don't have to be raw, cooked works too as long as you don't overdo it. Cut down on my favourite, cheese sauce on veggies. Definitely go for good cancer fighting veggies like broccoli, brussel sprouts, kale, other cruciforms and non-root vegetables generally. Choose different colours of veggies, green, orange, red. Substitute sweet potatoes for white potatoes. Create a list of your allowable foods before you go to the grocery store.

3. Increase the cancer fighting fruits such as blueberries, raspberries, pomegranate, citrus, read books identified in the resource section,appendix two for a more advice.

4. Eliminate what my mother has always said was poison, white sugar, high fructose corn syrup, etc. Research that blames sugars for a rise in cancer proliferation in Western Society has been available for years. Cancer cells like sugar, we don't want them to grow so cut the sugar, candy, sweetened chocolate (the unsweetened is apparently good).

5. Grains and fibre will help those who suffer from colon cancer. They are good for all for a variety of reasons.

6. Food sensitivity is apparently another epidemic in the modern world. The problem is that allergies and sensitivities cause stress in the body and stress reduces your immunity. Lowered immunity means the cancer has a better chance of establishing itself and surviving in your body. My advice is to invest in your health and pay to get tested for allergies through a blood test, then act on the results.

Food Planning

Our approach can be summarized as follows:

1. Research reliable sources on the internet, buy books recommended by your "health team". Books such as "Foods that Fight Cancer" by the Canadian team of Beliveau and Gingras. No, we are not getting paid to advertise, this is a great book.
2. Get tested for food intolerances and allergies. My naturopath was extremely helpful. If you have access to a nutritionist/nutritional counsellor or dietician, confer with them.
3. Using the above information create a listings of different kinds of food:
   - *Foods to avoid due to allergies/ intolerance/ sensitivities*
   - *Foods known to be cancer promoting (e.g. desserts containing sugar)*
   - *Foods with empty calories (potato chips, chocolate bars, etc.).*
   - *Recommended amount of water to drink daily to flush the system.*
   - As you might imagine the 'no fly" list was huge.
4. We then created our good list:
   - Foods that fight cancer
   - The *recommended amount of water to drink daily to flush the system.*

Originally the foods that fight cancer list seemed very foreign. There were things on that list, like Kale and Swiss Chard that we had no idea how to cook, the internet provided recipes.

Nobody had answered my basic question;

"If eating certain foods with toxins in them can help to trigger cancer, does eliminating toxins from your diet stop the triggering and slow or eliminate the cancer?"

The unifying theory would tell us that taking away a stressor should help. In addition eating foods that have been proven to prevent cancer will slow its progress if not stop it in its tracks.

What happened to that Japanese guy we talked about earlier who left Japan and came to North America and got cancer, did it go away when he moved back to Japan? Why don't we know the answer to such basic questions given the huge investment in the war on cancer since it was declared in1971.

Perhaps the governments that are dealing with the fallout from health care inflation should start researching topics like this that might reduce chronic disease and the demand for healthcare services.

There is a huge amount of information showing that certain foods fight cancer, do your research. In the NIH and other free search engines enter the following: food and cancer. Now substitute the specific food you are interested in for "food".

In conclusion, drink enough water, avoid processed foods and foods with toxins in them, read the labels on every thing you buy to ensure the foods you are buying are healthy choices, exercise to help the body flush the toxins out.

Food is medicine or poison. Poison is a negative stress, negative stress hurts your bodies ability to do gene repair, to have a healthy immune system and creates an environment conducive to cancer cell proliferation. Food as medicine fights cancer and other diseases.

Make sure you are on the right side of this equation.

CHAPTER FIVE - Keep Moving

"Walking is the best medicine"

Hippocrates

If you review the studies on exercise and lifestyle change and the impact on cancer, most studies found that exercise, weight reduction, low-fat diet, and reduced alcohol intake were associated with a decreased risk of cancer.

As one of the people we interviewed said "

"OK, this shouldn't be happening!"

"Why can't a diet of bacon cheeseburgers, fries and beer fight cancer? Why can't being a pizza eating, couch potato fight cancer? Life is not fair."

Apparently the proof is very clear, exercise does fight cancer. It would be nice if this was a conspiracy by the people trying to sell us a gym subscription, but sadly there is no evidence of that.

As George said *" I am not an athlete by nature. Weight has always been a challenge for me, too much not too little! I enjoy a slow walk through nature, sailing, a slow paddle in a kayak. Notice that slow is an adjective that is very prominent in my vocabulary about exercising. Really, I can take or leave exercise.*

The problem is that athletes, who are dominant in the industry from weight training gym's to yoga studios, have difficulty understanding couch potatoes.

In my case, my legs are long, my arms short, so in gym my legs used to catch on the pommel horse and you can imagine what happened next, face plant. I cannot touch my toes. The gym teacher laughed, but there again, he was a mean child torturing monster! This aversion to exercise is something I am trying to change, and kicking my addiction to being a couch potato is something that seems to be harder for me than quitting smoking was!

Unfortunately there is no legal pill you can take that suddenly makes you full of energy and eager to be athletic. With our luck it would probably have devastating side effects anyway.

Exercise is something that the recently diagnosed cancer patient needs to consider very carefully. Hard exercise can be stressful and if you are already in a weakened state you need to be careful. That is why experts recommend soft "restorative" exercise until you become stronger.

Soft exercise means restorative yoga, tai chi, chi kung, and slow no impact exercise such as walking. Find a cool place to walk like the forest, or by a lake.

David the pastor tells us;

"I started three tai chi classes a week after a month, and I was back in the gym after two months. I lost a lot of weight (but have gained it all back, I'm afraid). My blood pressure was normal until a week after I returned to work, which tells me something about my work. If you do all your exercises and many more (I can't recommend Tai Chi enough for this) and you have good fortune, you will not suffer much in the way of incontinence, but don't be so manly as to not wear pads— and don't send your wife to get them because she'll get the wrong kind (who needs 'wings' anyway?)—and don't let yourself get caught up short because when you have to go you will have to go now!" (David is a prostate cancer buddy).

Note, restorative yoga is slow not fast or hot, listen to your body, do only as much as feels comfortable. As my yoga instructor tells me, don't strain, breathe into the part of your body that feels like it is stretching. Athletes have perfectly proportioned bodies, no fat to speak of, lots of energy to spare. It is hard to identify with that type of person when you have struggled with weight all your life.

Unfortunately the research tells us to get over it. Do exercise daily. No, I am not kidding, this is actually important.

As a Tai Chi instructor I found that there is a group of people who worked mainly with their heads, academics, office workers and individuals who didn't move their body very much (for example truck drivers and factory workers who didn't have to move around a lot). These individuals were often out of touch with their body. They had trouble moving certain muscles, often had body pain, especially in their back and neck.

All these individuals gained much from re-establishing a link to their body and becoming more in tune with their bodily needs. Exercise really helps, but doing Tai Chi once a week isn't enough. Research has proven that we need to exercise every day.

We Need To Exercise Every Day

My dog Logan apparently knows this. Ever since I was diagnosed, his intensity of getting my attention to take him out has increased markedly. Ok, perhaps he always wanted to go for a walk and I had become really good at ignoring him.

Logan is a Westie, a white haired scottish terrier. To get me to walk he will roll over, sit on his hind legs and paw the air with his front paws and he actually talks to me, sort of a half growl, half whine (I should put him on you tube). Being totally anthropomorphic for a moment, he really seems to think his job is to get me moving. He does a good job.

Michigan researchers have found that dog owners are 34% more likely to meet the federal guidelines for exercise than other people, so Logan deserves credit. Get rid of your cat and get a dog, just joking about the cat, but not about the dog. Go to the local pound and rescue a cute one. A good piece of advice a friend gave me is to go for the bold one, the dog that comes forward to greet you. Not that the other dogs don't need saving, they do, but the bold one will not be shy about communicating his or her desire to go for a walk.

Walk half an hour to an hour every day. Push yourself gently to go faster, longer. Unless you got yourself a dog that is vertically challenged, the dog will easily out-walk and outrun you.

Exercise daily, rain or shine, snow or sleet. Just keep warm and keep moving. In our area the local hockey rink has a walking track that keeps us out of the worst weather. We walk every day. No excuses, well actually there are a million excuses, but we are learning to ignore them and go anyway.

That feeling of wanting to be a couch potato is not unique to you. From 60 to 96 percent of cancer patients, including those in remission report fatigue. I am a member of that club, unfortunately.

Research tells us that gentle exercise is very effective at reducing the amount of cancer related fatigue. This is one of those situations where you need to do the opposite of what you feel like doing. You feel tired, so you want to lay around, wrong! You feel tired, have a short nap then go and ride your bike, walk to the store and walk right past the tobacco and sweets! Go for the cancer fighting foods.

Inspire yourself, look at the You tube movies of the soldiers who lost limbs and still exercise like athletes. Set minor steps to achieve for each day or week, one more length of the pool, one more lap around the walking track, one more repetition of the weight at the gym. Try to push yourself just a little each week.

Yoga has always been interesting to me, but not the physical Hatha variety. My interest was always in Raja Yoga, Patanjali Yoga, Kriya Yoga, any Yoga that involved meditation but didn't involve what seemed to me to be contortions and slightly ridiculous looking physical exercise. Something about Yoga intrigued me enough to keep coming back every few years.

The need for physical exercise to beat the odds with cancer re-sparked an interest in the more physical varieties of Yoga. My good friends in Vancouver; Padma (of Padma TV fame) and Gary and Radha Bello have been very helpful in this regard. Liz and I have gone on their Yoga retreats to try to get me in something other than an apple or pear shape.

Initially I felt useless at it, even though my balance was good from Tai Chi and some aspects of flexibility weren't bad, some parts of me just didn't seem to work the way they needed to. I got over it. Fortunately they were kind enough not to laugh at my efforts.

After several months of off and on attempts at starting physical yoga on a regular basis I now feel like I am beginning to get there. My flexibility and energy levels have both increased gradually, frustratingly gradually. If you are out of shape, and I don't mean just fat, I mean inflexible in any way, Yoga will help you.

Now before I start sounding goofy like a recent convert, my advice is to get a good Yoga DVD and try doing it daily. Elizabeth and I have gone from Yoga once or twice a year (no kidding) to once a week, twice a week and now, we usually manage about five times per week. It is now at the point where we miss it if we miss a couple of days. It is hard to believe it took so long to get to this point and that I had been so out of touch with parts of my body. Resources we have found helpful are listed in Appendix 2.

There have been many times that I just wanted to go back to bed, watch the TV or just lie on the beach but Logan and Liz encouraged me to get up and out. Apparently they were right, keep moving!

"There's An APP For That!"

Become the master of the short nap. Research by NASA, the FAA and others have found that alertness increases with the short nap. There is some argument about the best length of a nap. Research shows that from 15 to 30 minutes is best, depending on which research you read. Longer naps run the risk of getting into deeper sleep which apparently makes you a little groggy for a while. So aim for the 15 to 20 minute nap. Believe it or not there really are "apps" for that. You can set the timer for the desired length of nap and your phone or other electronic device will wake you up. The issue is, when are they going to invent an "app" that recognizes when you are asleep then wakes you up 15 to 20 minutes later. No doubt someone is working on that!

Speaking of timers, one way to reduce the couch potato time and improve the exercise time is to put a PVR on your TV. Decide on the shows you are going to watch, record them, don't surf to find something to fill your time. Willpower is apparently both a hereditary and a learned behaviour. You can work on improving that willpower, but in the mean time, use technology! The less chance you have to sit on your couch the better. TV is addictive and the plot lines are so predictable. There are well over 200 TV channels and few worth watching. Remember, for the time you do allow yourself for watching the TV, choose comedy, laughter really is the best medicine for beating the odds. Subscribe to the comedy channel and comedy movies, leave the news and horror movies for another day.

Another alternative is to try one of the game attachments for your TV that have exercise games, dancing programs, etc. These will help you move in the house and will get you off the couch too.

Another tip for those of us that have to spend time at the computer, get a stand up desk. Mine is like an elevated table with shelves underneath. A high stool allows me to sit when my legs get tired, but mostly I stand.

An added bonus, studies have proven time and time again that bone density in cancer patients is significantly improved by taking the right supplements and exercising. As far as bone density is concerned, aerobics is best if you have recovered enough to do it, walking and yoga like exercise is second best, but just keeping moving works too. Research says to improve bone density, exercise and take vitamin D with your calcium supplements.

Aerobic exercise is apparently really important, a recent University of California study found that "over 180 various genes known to play a role in fighting cancer were more active when study participants exercised vigorously for more than three hours a week." We want that working for us to help beat the odds.

Yoga

Before we proceed, let me assure you that I do not own shares in a Yoga studio, but as a convert I can be like that guy who just quit smoking. That being said, there are some interesting facts you should know. Yoga researchers have found some very interesting results.

They have found that Yoga has a very positive health effect, beyond what you would expect from what appears to be simple stretching exercises. The mechanism is thought to be related to the protective chemicals released during Yoga poses which help the gene repair process work effectively and improve the immune system. Yoga has been shown to:

- Affect those genes related to increasing white blood cells,
- Improve the bodies response to antioxidants,
- Boost the immune and gene repair systems,
- Improve flexibility, strengthen muscles and reduce weight around the waist.

Reports are that Yogi's live longer, there is anecdotal evidence, but we couldn't find any evidence based studies to support this longevity claim. Further research in this area is needed. If the results show that Yogi's really do live longer and are less likely to get cancer then we will have another key to understanding cancer prevention.

One area that does seem to have some very promising research is yogic breathing. This breathing method is often known as pranayama; prana is sanskrit for life force, pranayama means extension of the life force. This set of breathing techniques has been shown to:

- reduce blood pressure,
- improve quality of life for people with asthma,
- reduce the symptoms of depression,
- help with post traumatic stress disorder and
- reduce the feelings of back pain.

How pranayama works at the cellular level is still unclear but studies have shown that antioxidant levels are better maintained, and individuals report improved breathing, reduction in fatigue and improved pain control. Considering it is almost free (buy a DVD if studio lessons are out of your financial reach) and takes only time, it is hard to see why everyone doesn't practice both yoga, pranayama and meditation. If you have cancer it is a no brainer. Really, get off the couch, do some restorative yoga, practice some yogic breathing, turn off the TV and meditate.

Once you have recovered from the treatments and have practiced restorative Yoga, Tai Chi, or walking for a while (daily!) you may want to try other forms of exercise. Try engaging in activities such as kayaking, canoeing, tennis, gentle weight lifting, jogging, more vigorous Yoga. Just ensure you pick something you enjoy and will continue to practice.

There have been some interesting studies that show that even ten minutes of exercise a day is better than none and that more than 25 minutes a day is best. Intensity isn't as important as getting out there and doing something. That being said, if you can do some aerobic exercise daily as mentioned previously it is cancer fighting.

One word of caution,as someone diagnosed with cancer you may want to stay away from areas that have heavy pesticide or fertilizer use such as Golf courses. Golf is great exercise (if you walk!) but the exposure to the chemicals can cancel out the good effects of the exercise.

Geoffrey's personal experience has been that routine is very important, it really helps him to stop rationalizing why he doesn't need to exercise that day. Here is his routine:

- Morning- meditation followed by Yoga.
- Aerobic exercise on the elliptical machine
- Afternoon- nap followed by long walk
- Evening-meditation, reading, perhaps some other activity such as dancing.

He tells us that if he is lucky enough to be invited to a warm climate he swims. His daily routine involves about an hour of exercise on average and at least 30 minutes per day, otherwise he reports that he actually feels fat.

Geoffrey reports that if a stressful event arises he may meditate and exercise more. His constant battle is weight gain, it is a side effect of the chemotherapy he is given, but more exercise keeps the weight constant, even more exercise causes weight loss.

His new regime is now possible three years after diagnosis only because the anemia and chronic fatigue from the cancer treatment has subsided somewhat. He reports that he cannot push it too much, even after three years, hopefully you are different.

In conclusion, a low level of fitness is a strong predictor of early death (Blair 2004). Exercise reduces symptoms of depression, diabetes and heart disease. Exercise helps to fight cancer, gives you more energy, we need energy to deal with disease and boost our immune systems, aerobic exercise stimulates gene repair. So please no excuses.

CHAPTER SIX - Treatment Options

The late twentieth century saw an explosion of information becoming available to everyone through computerization and the availability of the internet. These advances have given individuals with a disease unprecedented access to information about their disease and the current treatment modalities. These advances mean that most individuals who choose to become informed will become active participants in their healthcare decision making.

To participate in your healthcare decision making you need to do your due diligence and gather knowledge about your disease and the treatment options available to you.

With this knowledge (see Chapter One) you are ready to participate in making the decision about which course of treatment you wish to pursue.

David the Pastor continues....

"Naturally I had to investigate other options, and went off to see a radiologist. I was greeted by a big strapping young man with red hair and a pink tie (fashion faux or what?) who went over my numbers with me. He talked at some length about the

parameters of his craft and where I fit in, and I talked comfortably with him, enjoying his ease of presence and light humour. I was all set to follow this course of treatment and simply glowed in how easy it would all be. Then, as I smiled, he set his clipboard down and started to expound to considerable length as to why, given my age and stage of life, surgery would be the most comprehensive option. As he spoke, this young man of considerable size, got further and further into my space, and fairly loomed inches from my nose as he finished a tirade of several minutes duration, finishing with the rather deflating remark that if I were his father, he would see I got the surgery.

I hadn't realized until that moment I was that old!

I don't mind saying that this was the first time I felt frightened, and almost started crying (not a habit of mine). Then he started again, and I gently said, "You're a little close, and I heard every word you said." He realized that passion had got the best of *him and sat back, somewhat embarrassed I think. Susan and I drove home and scheduled the surgery.*

So we went back to the urologist, that kind but somewhat humourless man. He walked into the office and asked, "So, how are you?" "Haven't you heard?" I asked. "Heard what?" he said, looking alarmed. "Why, I have cancer!" I said. The briefest of smiles passed over his face. "Your right," he said, "stupid question.""

Choices

In some types of cancer diagnoses choosing treatment options is easy. This usually happens where treatment is almost 100% effective and a cure is almost guaranteed. This makes the treatment decision easy. In this situation why would anyone consider an alternative? May all of us in "the club nobody wanted to join" be so lucky.

One dramatic example is the new treatment for CML (chronic myelogenous leukemia). As explained to me by my friend who has worked in this field for many years, the results are almost miraculous. CML is diagnosed when normal white blood cells have chromosomal mutations and form abnormal white blood cells. These cells eventually start to crowd out normal cells with unfortunate results. A new drug treatment, actually a new class of drugs, targets the proteins created by the mutation. This treatment is not without side effects, some serious, so it is not for everyone. Those who are fortunate not to have life threatening side effects can be successfully treated with the new drugs.

Clinicians have found that the CML cancer goes into ***total remission*** for ten or more years with this drug treatment, remarkable. ***There are no detectable symptoms*** during this period! There has been a similar result with the designer drug Herceptin when used to treat certain types of breast cancer. Not all designer drugs have been so clearly effective. A drug for advanced prostate cancer for example,which is a vaccine has stimulated a lot of controversy, even though it was approved by the FDA.

Researchers hope that gene based research will allow the creation of other drugs that are able to create total remission in other cancers too. A lofty goal, but one that will take time.

The Rest Of Us

So, for those of us who have diagnoses that don't have a miraculous drug cure, or for those of us who don't have insurance and cannot afford to buy the miraculous drugs, ***what do we do in the interim?***

Without the miracle drug option there are few therapies that are easy, inexpensive, pain free or 100% effective. So you have to make a choice, or a series of choices. There are few situations or conditions where a choice must be made yesterday, so take the time to decide how you will proceed.

"We drove to Barrie, a town 30 minutes away, to see a radiation oncologist about the possibility of Fred doing a course of radiation treatment in an effort to prolong his life by a few months. The upshot is that the doctor thinks the tumour is too large (she said it was the size of a basket ball) to use radiation to target things with great accuracy; right now it would do more harm than good. However, he has been approved for an experimental drug that blocks how cancer cells dispose of their waste, killing the cell. He will start that pill tomorrow, and see what happens. Best case scenario, it might shrink the tumour to a size where radiation could be used down the road. Keep your fingers crossed!"

Keep your fingers crossed indeed.

Without a cure we are left to beat the odds using a mixture of common sense, good research and good help from our friends, relatives and our dream team we have assembled to help us.

Considering Your Options

The first and most effective way of starting to evaluate options is to ask each member of your health team the key question *"what would you (your health advisor) do if they were you?"*. By team we mean the extended version of your health team including everyone who is helpful regardless of their credentials. Gone are the days when you just ask your doctor, if you want to beat the odds.

Remember, the average life expectancy for your diagnosis was set mainly by people who just listened to their doctor, so push the envelope and ask all your health team. There is no harm in gathering other opinions. Here again is the key question;

"what would they do if they were you?"

While it seems like a simple question, it is not, they are not you. Many health professionals don't like answering this question. What is so effective about this question is that some health professionals have not put themselves in their patient's shoes. The very act of doing so can cause them to stop reacting and giving pat answers and really put themselves in your place and consider their answer.

In my case the answers from the medical and non-medical side were the same, so initially it was an easy decision.

If you have a diverse team, as is recommended in chapter three and you have a complex health issue, then you may have several answers. If this is the case, the next step is to filter the cultural, professional and individual bias of the person giving a response.

Although we don't like to admit it, each profession has a built in bias that results from their training and the cultural memes in their professional group. Medical doctors have been trained to offer solutions that are surgical, radiation or drug (chemotherapy) based. Naturopaths lean towards supplements, herbs, allergies and diet related solutions. If you are fortunate to have a nutritionist on your team they are diet focussed.

Your favorite Aunt who drives you to your cancer treatment may have had a bad experience with a type of treatment or a certain professional. Consider what she says carefully, is she biased? Did she really understand the science behind the treatment received? Often individuals cannot bear to admit that a loved one died naturally, or at least died because there was nothing anyone could do. This is especially so if the individual is depressed or just a negative person. There again, your aunt and her opinion could be right. How do you know? Almost everyone has a bias from their experiences and training, so to counter this we need to rely on evidence based research when feasible.

Consider all the options and the advice carefully. Most importantly, do your due diligence research as outlined in chapter one, or get your friend who is good with the internet to help you do the research.

Remember, start with the evidence based research:

- First, what options are there?
- What options does medical research recommend?
- What other viable options are there?
- What are the outcomes of each?
- How good is the research source?
- Is the evidence reproducible?
- What are the side effects?
- Does the suggested treatment warrant the risk of side effects?

These are huge questions. Involve your whole team in the evaluation process. How much effort you put into this will obviously depend on how serious your diagnosis is, how invasive the treatment options are, the seriousness of the side effects and the projected outcomes. Clearly, if this is a curable cancer with little risk you won't need to spend as much time evaluating the options as someone with non-curable cancer combined with other complex diseases.

Alternatives

Evaluate the next level of options, less evidence based, but perhaps for good reason (remember no patent, no profit, no research!). Do you feel comfortable with any of those options, ask the same questions, what are the outcomes, side effects, etc.

You now need to make a decision. In my case we decided that the medical option was feasible and that the side effects were reasonable, that being said however, our research also helped us to decide that many of the naturopathic options were also of added benefit and some would reduce the side effects of the cancer treatment I was receiving without reducing their effectiveness.

In fact when I asked the naturopaths what they would do in my case, they recommended the medical option with supplemental help from certain items they recommended. I was really pleased by their response. Their advice confirmed the research that we had undertaken. Their advice was very helpful, as mentioned elsewhere in this book, their suggestions during radiation were effective, in addition they recommended some evidence based supplements. All of the supplements they recommended were supported by good evidence based research.

Clearly my personal bias against Naturopaths had been misplaced, at least with the very professional group of naturopaths that I met through the Naturopathic college. My experience does not extend beyond that. Consequently, my advice is to be cautious until the worth of each individual health professional is proven.

Don't let your biases kill you. A good friend of mine died early of cancer because he rejected naturopathic advice and believed the doctors prognosis (to the week). Also, my beautiful young sister probably died early because she rejected the medical treatment option and "went all natural". Bias either way can kill you, so keep an open mind. Naturopaths report seeing many people who reject medical advice and refuse to listen when the Naturopath advises them to see a medical doctor.

Please approach your cancer with a good dose of common sense. Just because one medical doctor (or naturopath, or other health professional) has been rude to you or treated you badly in the past does not mean they are all wrong or that any research is totally wrong.

Suspend your disbelief of medicine or alternative medicine and combine them to create the unique comprehensive combination of treatment that is best for you.

Some health professionals get stuck with professional blinders on which make them unable to see beyond their profession's bias. Like the old psychology study, give a man a hammer and his whole world becomes a search for nails, even where nails aren't the best solution.

Surgery is one area that has received much criticism for over use. Studies in the US recently for example have shown that 30% of breast biopsies were surgical and the standard is 10% (the majority are done by needle biopsy which is less invasive, safer and cheaper).

David the Pastor continues...."So the big day arrived, Dec.1, 2010. Somewhere during the night two days before, a leak appeared in the bathtub and took out a big section of the kitchen ceiling. Some time a couple of weeks later my dog required surgery." What else could go wrong?" some folks might ask. Well...

don't. But sometimes that last straw never comes; it's all just grist for the mill when important events like this are taking place in such a personal forum. We drove to the hospital at 5:00 a.m., went through all the steps, suffered the four or five attempts at installing the I.V., then I kissed Susan and held her for a moment, then I headed to the O.R.

I was greeted by a bevy of busy nurses all asking me if I knew why I was here... an odd question to repeat five times, I thought. So when a very young, very pretty, and very exotically foreign anesthesiologist walked in and asked me, "Mr. Blank do you know why you're here?" I blurted out, "Oh my God! Don't you?"

The nurses started giggling, but she didn't understand the humour and was a little put out. I think it's probably a bad idea to piss off someone who's about to stick a four-inch needle into your spine, don't you? But by this time I was feeling a little in need of humour just to keep myself going, as I am not a brave man.

The young doctor, however, was a little flustered and kept talking without finishing her sentences. I looked at the obviously experienced O.R. nurse and smiled a fearful smile: "Does she realize that not finishing her sentences does nothing to inspire confidence?" I asked. She smiled broadly, but put her finger to her lips. "Sh!" she hissed, "behave!" I was having trouble achieving the necessary position for the proper application of a spinal block (some things we just don't have enough time to practice), and the doctor's voice was starting to sound impatient. The nurse leaned over me and took my head, whispered some directions, and moved my face straight into her chest. This would have pushed me into hilarity, except she knew what she was doing and this very personal moment was interrupted by the needle. Then things started getting... calmer, much, much calmer. The last thing I remember was the face of my very kind and competent surgeon leaning over me and asking, "Do you have any other questions before we start?" "Yes," said I, "is this like with tonsils, and can I have *the little bugger in a jar?" He did not laugh. But the nurse did. And then I was asleep.*

Truthfully I don't think I want the folks with the knives and big needles to have much humour. I want them to be serious, and very, very good at what they do. But not everyone should get off so easy."

A recent breakthrough in surgical techniques was recently developed called colour coded surgery. This new technique uses fluorescent colouring to clearly show cancer cells in the surgical field by making them fluorescent. The surgeon can be very sure that she/he removed all the cancer cells using this technique. A further expansion of this approach also colour codes nerves as a different colour and minimizes potential nerve damage. Ask if this new technique is available in your area.

Radiation is another way of killing cancer cells but with a shotgun approach, good cells die with the cancer cells and it is traumatic to the body. A long time cancer researcher and good friend calls radiation treatment for cancer as the equivalent of the carpet bombing of Dresden during the second world war. The armed forces were destroyed, but so were the museums, art galleries and sculptures, not to mention the "collateral damage", the women and children. Although he further went on to say that in the absence of better options it is often the best option.

Modern radiation therapy has advanced significantly over time, the radiation therapists are able to focus the equipment much more accurately than in the past so less damage is done, unfortunately there is usually some "collateral damage" to healthy tissue. The extent of the damage depends on how small the tumor is and where in the body it is located. Sometimes radiation is the better medical alternative. Recent trials of surgically placing sources of radiation next to tumours has also proven to be quite effective with certain cancers.

My personal choice was for radiation rather than surgery since the cancer had escaped the organ where the cancer initiated. Even though some collateral damage was to be expected, it was the alternative projected to have the most positive outcome. Everyone agreed that it was the best option for my cancer at that time.

Sometimes several techniques in combination (e.g. surgery, radiation and chemo) are prescribed. Do your research. If radiation is your option, I would strongly recommend seeing a naturopath. They will be able to recommend supplements, creams and probiotics that will help to reduce the impact of radiation without reducing the effectiveness of the treatment itself.

Chemotherapy is another way of either killing cancer cells or shutting down the blood vessels supplying the cancer cells and thus starving them. Certain chemotherapy solutions are like carpet bombing too, they may be very traumatic. Others are more subtle, the chemo I have taken for several years to shrink the tumour was quite effective. Unfortunately, the side effects of the drugs didn't become evident for almost a year and eventually became so bothersome that we had to consider giving it up due to the severity of the side effects.

To give up the treatment was a trade off decision, was I willing to risk the cancer becoming rampant again, or was I willing to accept the side effects that could also potentially kill me? Further investigation revealed that the side effects were worth suffering through. Later on further research emerged that showed that one suspected side effect, heart issues was in fact not an issue. This underlines the fact that we need to continue monitoring the research to ensure that the alternative course we are on is still the best.

What are the odds, what does the medical literature say? Do your research.

Supplements and herbs are often a gentler approach to what is essentially chemotherapy. The decision to go this route alone is a difficult one because the evidence that supports these treatments is not "gold standard" research.

Some people are so "anti" the medical establishment they abandon it and go completely "natural". As mentioned earlier this is a topic that needs serious consideration. As a first line of defense natural methods are seldom the best option in a very serious case of cancer, but in some less virulent forms natural methods may be very effective. A friend managed to treat their mild case of skin cancer with natural methods only.

The Naturopathic College assigned a very bright student to my case. She provided extensive proof of her recommendations, and as I mentioned earlier I was really surprised by the fact that much of the naturopathic work was very scientific and well documented in "good" medical journals. Some was even peer reviewed research and while not the $100 million "gold standard" double blind clinical research it was the next best thing.

This really surprised me. Clearly I had been listening to too much to the misinformation about naturopaths being circulated by non believers who prefer to ignore facts..

The obvious question that came to mind was "why doesn't the medical profession work more closely with naturopaths?".

During my radiation therapy the naturopath stopped me taking certain naturopathic supplements that were known to reduce the effectiveness of the radiation. In addition, the naturopaths recommended salves to take away the burning feelings one gets from radiation. Being repeatedly radiated over one area of the body causes burning sensations in the skin, it actually turns red, the salves really helped. The naturopaths also recommended herbal drinks to take away the internal burning sensations. These were very effective. Most importantly they recommended that I take powerful probiotics to reestablish my internal gastric bacteria that had been destroyed by the radiation after each session. These were prescribed to help with digestion. The radiation centre staff doctors and nurses had recommended an over the counter drug for indigestion.

Unfortunately patients expect a drug prescription from the medical staff as a solution. Naturopaths alternatively tend to recommend remedies based on biological function. In too many areas, medicine seems to have moved away from the original approach of trying to remedy the whole person and has replaced that with treating the symptoms with drugs. Sir William Osler would not be happy.

Studies have clearly indicated that a large percentage of cancer patients will visit both medical and naturopathic professions. For the most part they will not discuss what their naturopath recommended with those on the medical side of the fence.

Anyone who has been in the health system as a patient and has tried to raise the possibility of seeing an alternative medicine practitioner with their medical practitioner knows the situation well. The usual response according to most patients I talked with, was that they were ridiculed or looked down on by the medical practitioner, so they learned to say nothing. This needs to change.

Side Effects

One area you will need to spend some extra time on is the side effects issue. Side effects are often listed differently in different places.

Jules had read the insert in the drug package but it wasn't until she fell that she raised the question of side effects with her team. She was told by the pharmacist that a certain very serious side effect was rare. On a more detailed search for drug side effects it turned out that the so called "rare" side effect had a frequency of one in one hundred patients. Jules it turned out was one of those "rare" cases. The result was that she almost died from the side effect. She collapsed on the sidewalk and had to be taken to hospital.

This type of situation happens more often when more than one physician is dealing with a case. Her comment was "one in a hundred seems pretty frequent to me, doesn't it to you? How many millions of patients are on this drug? How many are having these brutal side effects and being ignored as I was? How many died?"

Good point Jules, falling on the sidewalk would be the cause of death listed, not the drug that caused the fainting spell. Serious and poorly documented side effects are not an isolated situation for people with more than one disease, a fairly common thing these days. For example, an individual with cancer is seeing an oncologist but they are may also be seeing a cardiologist for a heart issue, an endocrinologist for diabetes and their family doctor who is treating them for other health issues. These health professionals are not always aware of what the others are prescribing, even though in a perfect world they should be.

Some pharmacists will catch potential drug interaction issues, in the case of Jules both the doctors and pharmacist missed it, even the doctor who was checking out her symptoms in emergency missed the fact that this was a drug side effect. So take charge and check out what all the side effects are of the drugs you have been prescribed.

Peter's friend tells us of his mother,

"She was on 16 different drugs from five separate physicians. The dementia was ruining her life, it went away when we started asking questions that resulted in 10 prescriptions being discontinued. Nobody had been monitoring the drug interactions, or the fact that many of the prescriptions were for the same treatment but prescribed by different doctors. This was patient abuse by neglect."

Until good computer systems with electronic health records and intelligent systems are in place everywhere to catch such interactions, make sure that you research each drug you are prescribed, individually, for side effects.

In conclusion, do your due diligence, get the opinions from all team members, sleep on it, then proceed with your chosen treatment option.

CHAPTER SEVEN - Spontaneous Remission

A review using the National Institute of Medicine's search engine; Pub Med , revealed 8,800 articles on spontaneous remissions in clinical journals . Most of these articles were anecdotal and as such did not represent solid evidence based research. That being said, the fact that there were 8,800 articles on this topic is pretty telling that this is something we need to be paying attention to.

Remission means that your cancer symptoms have gone away, at least for the present. The previously mentioned new drugs that affect gene mutations have been known to result in remission. For the most part however, other attempts at trying to purposefully create remission have not had as much success. Well to be fair, in scientific terms they have not had consistent replicability and so scientists have been skeptical enough to say they don't work. Applying science this rigidly may be causing us to throw out the baby with the bath water.

As the cases in the NIH search-engine show, the phenomena known as spontaneous remission, or as many call it "miracles" are well documented and if you are fortunate, you may become such a case.

Before we move on, let us address the concept of "miracles".

My friend Bill has outlived the doctors who told him he had two years to live, twenty five years ago. He swears that religious miracles do exist. He will tell you that prayer caused a miracle and killed his cancer.

Neb tells me that her husband took her to Lourdes in France and her energy returned, something that had gone after the chemotherapy.

As Susan tells in another example..." Hope came in the form of a fellow patient who had gone into "spontaneous remission" as the oncologists labeled it. We called it a miracle. James and Mary were religious, they listened eagerly as the patient offered hope, something that the doctors had surgically removed with their clinically cold responses. Suddenly life seemed worth living again. The dark pall that is cancer slowly disintegrated in the light of hope. James grew visibly taller as the conversation continued. Mary decided to learn more about embracing healing and allowing God to do the heavy lifting. A burden was lifted from her shoulders."

Miraculous things do occur, religious individuals believe in them, atheists and many scientists say it is just an issue of the underlying science not being fully understood. One side calls them miracles, the other spontaneous remission. Each group on either side of this discussion is adamant and so there is little to be gained from regurgitating their arguments. That is a debate for another book, so we will set it aside.

Epidemiology And Spontaneous Remission

Epidemiologists are professionals who study the statistics of disease, such as the incidence of cancer, or the correlation between an environmental toxin in food and the incidence of a certain type of cancer. Epidemiological study requires great patience and the ability to analyze data. If there is no data, there is no study. This is a huge issue where the relevant data has not been collected.

"Gold standard" epidemiological studies of spontaneous remission do not exist because the data is very difficult to obtain. If you have remission you drop out of the mainstream health system so data collection systems have no idea whether you moved, got better or died. They also have no idea about all those people who decide not to use the mainstream health care system in the first place.

One meets quite a number of such people at the naturopathic clinic and spiritual healing centres. Similarly there are individuals who use both medical and alternative medical treatments and don't let the medical system know. We don't tend to track them either.

There are some studies being started now that will over time consider some of these factors. Such studies follow populations of individuals over time, so the results typically take many years to emerge.

Remission is so poorly studied that the statistical estimates in the mainstream literature vary from 1 in 5 cases to 1 in 140,000 cases. Seriously, one study actually claimed that 1 in 5 cases of breast cancer go into remission naturally. There is no really solid data to confirm or deny this.

The bottom line is that we know remission occurs "naturally", we don't know how and we really don't know how often that happens. We know that remission occurs because we have actual medical evidence (biopsies, blood tests, imaging, studies that confirm remission), but because we cannot replicate it we generally ignore that proof.

An interesting Toronto study of 200 survivors of ovarian cancer (7 years on average beyond diagnosis) found that women who were in remission attributed their lack of cancer recurrence to:

- positive attitude (82.5%),
- close medical follow-up (82.0%),
- healthy lifestyle (69.0%),
- prayer (68.0%),
- stress reduction (66.5%),
- diet (63.0%), and

- exercise (58.5%).

Most survivors reported healthy behaviors with respect to not smoking (95.5%), balanced diet (92.0%), and regular exercise (65.0%).

Of note was that 82% took vitamins or other supplements.

How many of them shared this information with their physician is unknown.

As previously mentioned, most of the people we met at a naturopathic clinic kept the fact that they took supplements, vitamins and even saw a naturopath to themselves because they feared ridicule from their doctors. This fear of ridicule prevented patients from sharing dietary changes, talking about yoga, meditation and other stress reduction techniques they were implementing. One oncologist we talked with claimed, contrary to the evidence, that vitamins, supplements and negative stress played no part in helping to fight cancer! People believe what they want to, regardless of the facts, including some doctors.

What causes remission/ regression/ miracles depends on what you believe. If you are a scientist, it is an undocumented chemical reaction. If you are religious it is an intervention by God. If you are a believer in drinking apple cider vinegar, it is apple cider vinegar. Until there is proof we need to counsel individuals on all sides of this discussion to be open minded and encourage those who run the health systems to begin to document remission more carefully.

It would seem reasonable and wise to research remission more seriously than we currently do, there may be inexpensive cures we are ignoring because not all relevant data is being collected. The terminal cancer patient really doesn't care what causes remission or regression as long as it happens.

All that being said there are a number of theories as to why spontaneous remission occurs.

- The most popular is that the immune system somehow is reset and starts keeping the cancer under control. This makes sense since we know that almost every cadaver that is tested for cancer has some cancer cells. Even those individuals who have never been diagnosed with cancer had cancer cells present. So clearly for people without a cancer diagnosis the body keeps the cancer cells under control and in people with a cancer diagnosis it doesn't.
- Another key finding is that the precursor to some people going into remission is a fever. This may be something resulting from an allergic reaction to an insect sting or simply a bad case of the flu. It seems that in the process of fighting this fever the body also recognizes cancer cells as the enemy and fights it too, remission ensues. The finding that a fever triggered an immune response to cancer has led to some weird and wonderful therapies such as raising the core body temperature to simulate a fever, inducing a fever using venom or another trigger.

Some people have reportedly entered remission in this way. Don't try this at home...

- Other theories are based on the viral or bacterial causation model. Some non-mainstream researchers believe that the cause of all cancer is an agent such as a bacteria or a virus. Research has shown that there are some established associations in some cancers. One type of bacteria has been shown in peer reviewed studies to cause stomach cancer. Hepatitis B and C viruses are implicated in some types of liver cancer. Young people are now being vaccinated against HPV known to cause cervical cancer. Originally all these were formerly thought to be triggered by genetics or a carcinogen, not bacteria or a virus. In these types of cases, antivirals or antibiotics as appropriate can be effective. There may be other forms of cancer with viral or bacterial links.
- Some cancer remission has been noted after individuals have been given antibiotics for the treatment of other diseases. More study is needed.
- Intravenous (IV) vitamin C at certain levels acts as an antiviral and a recent CMAJ study found that it also can kill cancer cells. Some cases of remission have been noted with IV vitamin C which was recently shown not to have side effects.
- Certain types of bowel cancer seems to respond to certain antibiotics. The mechanism is not really known.
- A theory was put forward by a Sloan Kettering physician, Dr Coley who died in 1936. He postulated that certain

bacteriological infections were the cause of remission. There were apparently 900 cases documented where he induced a fever by bacteriological infection. His first case experienced remission of throat cancer. While there were a number of remissions and many cases that improved the FDA eventually prevented him from continuing. The reason they gave was that the experiments were not always reproducible (that issue of replicability again) and some patients died of the fever that was induced.

This is another situation where further research would be warranted. Clearly we do not want patients dying of the treatment. That said however, we know the therapy was useful in certain cases, why not offer the testing with so called incurable cancer patients who are terminal and who volunteer?

Most of the huge body of research on spontaneous remission has looked at single anecdotal cases, here are some interesting ones culled from the National Institutes of Health database. Our purpose is not to suggest they are potential cures, simply interesting areas for future research. They are included here to stimulate further discussion:

✦The lung cancer patient who also had hypothyroidism and when injected with the thyroid drug the lung cancer went into remission. The thyroid drug increases the metabolic rate and this is thought to be what triggered the remission. This experiment was repeated with only "limited success" in other patients and was abandoned as a cure.

- ✦Apparently in the previous case, the original patient was also starving due to his condition and some believe this was an important component to remission. There are quite a number of other documented cases where starvation is present when the patient went into remission.
  Cancer cells grow at a very fast rate and need a lot of energy, considerably more than normal cells. Cancer cells actually build their own blood supply to deliver the energy to the growing cancer cells. Individuals who are starving don't have very much excess energy to offer the cancer cells.
- ✦The case of the man reportedly bitten by a "brown recluse" spider who went into remission as his body fought the venom. He survived the bite and his cancer went into remission.
- ✦The case of the child with an eye tumor who went into complete remission upon treatment with a gluten free diet. Allergies cause stress to the immune system, perhaps food allergies contribute to cancer or act as a component in the cancer triggering process. Allergies, like Asthma are certainly a form of stress and stress is cumulative and a cancer trigger.
- ✦Researchers working with several patients found that using a pulsed electrical field on skin melanomas caused complete remission in 7 weeks. Cancer cells are less complex than normal cells and more susceptible to death from energy fields such as radiation.

✦Researchers recently found that natural spontaneous remission in a certain type of liver cancer (HCC) occurred frequently. The spontaneous remissions were so frequent that they needed to be considered in clinical trials of drugs being tested to control the cancer. The higher frequency of natural remission made the drugs look more effective than they actually were.

✦A five year old girl with acute lymphoblastic leukemia went into remission following a fever and blood transfusion.

✦The16 year old patient with twice relapsed leukemia (AML) who achieved complete remission by treatment with Ayurvedic medicine. Ayurvedic medicine is thousands of years old and uses techniques considered strange to western medicine.

✦The documented case of a person with neck cancer going into remission after treatment with Reiki. Energy healing is a fascinating area with many thousands of documented "miracle" cures. Perhaps mind over matter, or maybe something we don't understand yet. There are a huge number of documented cases of Shamen, Spiritual Healers, Reiki Healers, and Therapeutic Touch Healers who have worked with individuals with cancer diagnoses and created or triggered spontaneous remission, or as they call it, miracles.

While the scientific community gives even less credibility to these cases many have been well documented by physicians. Harry Edwards, a spiritual healer from the United Kingdom had thousands of well documented cases of remission as did Edgar Cayce in the United States. Many medical doctors at the time provided evidence of cures, including x-rays and personal testimonials. Lourdes in France has 67 well documented “miracles”. While this doesn’t sound like a lot given the millions of visitors to Lourdes each year, the criteria for recognizing a miracle are very stringent. One of the criteria being evidence that no other treatment was provided. If we include the cases that medicine said were incurable and the treatment failed, then the patient visited Lourdes the number of miracles swells to the thousands.

Is this “mind over matter” or something science just doesn’t understand?

Much of this type of miraculous healing is available today, but is kept away from the media due to the aggressive threats by litigious non believers. Modern day spiritual healers need to be very careful that they aren’t sued for practicing “medicine”. The result is that much of their healing is called healing the spirit and is not documented for fear of legal action. (my favourite line from Shakespeare; Henry the Sixth, Part 2, Act 4 Scene 2)

Placebo

The placebo effect is where a cure occurs without the application of a treatment agent. In clinical trials individuals are assigned randomly to a group receiving the trial drug or to a group receiving a placebo. The placebo is often an intravenous saline solution, or a sugar coated pill, or some other "thing" that makes the patient think that they are receiving treatment. This is done since the placebo effect (people getting well with the placebo rather than any treatment) occurs occasionally. Some drugs are often proven no more effective than the placebo. In those cases the $100 million drug research is abandoned.

What happens to all those patients who were given a placebo who get well? Who keeps track of the patients who spontaneously recovered? There is no incentive for the drug companies to keep track of that information, but there is a huge advantage for society. We should be collecting that information then carefully studying it.

The placebo effect cures many people and we really don't understand why. The most common answer is that we believe it is the power of the human mind, mind over matter. More on this in chapter nine.

Science insists on "replicability", and in most applications of science, so it should. Another scientist should be able to copy the method used and see the same result. That seems to be an obvious requirement in medical research. It certainly is very important when considering drug research.

The question is should replicability be looked upon as an absolute necessity when it comes to research on such treatments as placebo, reiki and spiritual healing or are there just too many uncontrollable variables to insist on such rigor? We are told that energy based healing depends on the healers wellbeing as well as the patient. If an energy healer heals 20 out of thirty people, shouldn't that be considered good? If I were one of the 20 people I would think so. Yet tomorrow, that same energy healer may only help one person out of thirty. Should they be considered a failure? One statistic that has been noted with Reiki for example is that one third of the patients improve markedly, one third have reduction in symptoms and in one third there is no effect. One doctor friend laughed when he heard this and said that compared well with his results!

As a scientist my concern is that we are throwing the baby out with the bathwater because of the lack of consistency. Perhaps we just don't understand the science behind the phenomenon. Are we potentially missing a great opportunity by rejecting it out of hand because it doesn't meet the overly strict criteria we have today.

There is a risk for the research scientist studying such phenomena, that they will be labelled as flaky. The medical field is very competitive when it comes to research grants Appearing to be flaky can be a dangerous career move. The result is that few researchers volunteer to seriously study such topics and the money available for research is not substantial. On the other hand, in the field of $100 million per drug research, there is a lot of money and a guaranteed future. Clearly the research table is slanted in favour of drug research all the way around.

Science tries to control all variables except one to see if a treatment works. Clearly this is an intelligent approach. The problem is that this approach doesn't work when we don't have any idea what the contributing factors are.

Let us look at an example, we know that asbestos causes lung cancer, yet we also know that some individuals are resilient to exposure. Individuals with the same level of exposure will show varying results, some get cancer sooner than others, some get cancer and recover, some seem to be resilient and don't get cancer. Scientists hypothesize that this resilience is genetic, but we don't know for certain. It could just as easily be that we are more resilient due to our ability to handle stress, what our diet is, whether we exercise, etc.

We haven't studied every variable, for example,we don't know if resilient individuals ate more broccoli, or exercised more, or ate Brazil nuts daily (they are the richest source of selenium and several studies have shown a link between certain cancers and selenium deficiency).

All we know is that in populations exposed to asbestos at certain levels of exposure, a certain percentage of the people who are exposed died of lung cancer. This establishes the potential causality.

It is very difficult to design good studies to link cause and effect, remember our example, everyone who eats a tomato will die! The war on cancer has focussed too much on drug solutions and not enough on the causes and human resilience to cancer. We need to start focussing research on those who survive beyond the average.

It is only when we have really good data that we can prove causality beyond a doubt. The lack of good data initially was the reason the tobacco industry managed to successfully fight for so many years even after most people were convinced that tobacco triggered lung cancer. They kept dragging out those rare resilient individuals who smoked daily and lived to be 90.

Potential carcinogens require testing to see if they are cancer causing. Most of this research happens in the lab.The reason is that causality cannot be tested well in human experiments. This is because one needs to kill or maim the subjects. Researchers often use animals as human substitutes. In our example, they exposed rats to asbestos and repeatedly had a certain percentage of the population of rats die at certain levels of toxicity, that was considered a good way to prove causality. A causal link between asbestos and cancer was established.

Perhaps, the lack of replicability in the research of spontaneous remission should be looked at differently. Environmental exposure, resilience to stress, lack of important nutrients, exercise and other factors could easily explain differences in reactions of patients to carcinogens. Could it be that one miners love of broccoli (a known anti-oxidant) saved him from developing lung cancer while his friend standing next to him, getting the same exposure to asbestos hated vegetables and contracted lung cancer.

Resilience is not just genetic, it is also clearly a result of lifestyle, exposure to stress and the ability to handle stress.

The obsession with evidence based research (double blind, peer reviewed, replicable) is admirable. In a perfect world with endless supplies of research money it would be ideal. The problem is that it is not always realistic or even advisable when it only results in drug solutions to problems over alternatives that may be equally as viable and probably more affordable.

The no patent, no profit, no research solution of the medical industrial complex is apparently producing health systems that are too expensive and not necessarily as clinically effective as they might be. Drugs often have side effects that are unacceptable, yet we hold to them and ignore potentially viable alternatives due to lack of research funding.

What does all this mean to you, diagnosed with cancer and having been told that there is no easy cure. Clearly the wise course is to consider any alternative that isn't going to be harmful. In other words those alternatives and lifestyle changes discussed in this book.

Here is a simple story that illustrates how sometimes common sense solutions are better and cheaper, it was recounted by a friend who works part time in Cuba.

"Mel became ill as we were traveling through Cuba. When she got sick we went to a corner "green medicine" doctor. There are many of these local doctors all over Cuba. She was seen right away.

The doctor diagnosed dehydration, gave her a banana to eat and water to drink and told her to sit in the shade for a couple of hours and see if she was all right, she was. The banana replaced the electrolytes, the water rehydrated her, she was fine.

Now I ask you, compare the response we would have had in a developed country; ambulance called, transport to hospital emergency room, IV started, drugs given, held overnight for monitoring, discharged in morning, $Cha-ching, $ Cha-ching,!"

Sir William Osler would not be impressed, clearly as health professionals we have a responsibility to promote lower cost solutions when they are viable since we can then conserve resources for the patients who really need the expensive alternatives.

Are we too drug obsessed, have we talked ourselves into a path that really is not in our best interests? Clearly the answer is yes! How do we get out of this rut? The way out is to research the proven alternative methods outlined in this book, to compare drugs with alternatives as well as against a placebo.

In conclusion, whether we decide to try something that might trigger spontaneous remission should be up to us. Terminal patients should have the option of trying more risky alternatives. Most importantly, alternatives that have been shown to have no risk, have compelling evidence that they could reduce cancer incidence and help cancer sufferers extend their lives should be researched actively. That research should be funded by the government funded health systems that will benefit financially if less costly alternatives are found to be effective anticancer therapies.

CHAPTER EIGHT- Psychology - Stress

"A wise man should consider that his health is the greatest of human blessings and learn how, by his own thought, to derive benefit from his illnesses."

Hippocrates

David writes, as a Pastor who has heard many stories over the years

" I would say that most folks, when receiving the doctor's decree of cancer, freeze up in fear or flee into denial. Finally in August of 2010 my wife, Susan, the doctor and I sat down and he gave me the news. Whether it was my lack of imagination, my faith, or the many stories I'd heard in my work, I did not feel that sense of denial nor any fear. But I knew that this would be as much, or more, of a trial for Susan. My first response was to look at her and apologize! " It's not your fault," she said. But it *wasn't about blame. I felt regret for this interruption in our lives."*

We remember well the day a person walked on the moon and we remember well the day we became members of "the club nobody wants to join".

At this point the reader with a rigid science background may need to suspend their disbelief. What is discussed here is not necessarily peer reviewed, double blind, evidence based research from top shelf clinical research journals. The psychology of cancer diagnosis, treatment and recovery doesn't lend itself to such studies; nevertheless science indicates that overcoming the psychological trauma can help speed our recovery.

Blaming The Victim

It is easy for discussions of the psychological aspects of cancer to deteriorate into "blaming the victim". Most cancer victims have experienced the person who with complete insensitivity says "I wonder what you did to end up with cancer".

Some of the victim blaming comes from ancient sources. The Bible for example has passages where individuals are healed by having the apostle say "let your sins be forgiven" (e.g. Matthew 9:1-8). This is included simply to indicate how blaming the victim is not a new thing in society but an age old tradition.

Some people today still say that illness is due to something that the individual has done either in this life or if believers in reincarnation, even a past life.

This chapter is not intended to blame those diagnosed with cancer in any way. As the cancer theory in Appendix one indicates, cancer is triggered by multiple causes. Cancer is triggered by a combination of what we term stressors; pollution, psychological and/or physiological stress, contaminated food, and hereditary genetic issues. In some cases the stress we have may also have been affected by our past actions, but to argue that past actions are the only possible cause of illness is taking things too far.

So what exactly do we mean by stressors?

Stressors

Stress in this context is "negative stress", something that adversely affects the ***mind and/or the body***. The important point to remember is that ***stress is additive***. In other words, small stresses (psychological and physical) can build into a large stress load.

It is important to remember also that negative stress, both psychological and physical can also be reduced. This chapter is written to help the individual diagnosed with cancer to recognize their stress, reduce their negative stress levels and in so doing, increase their odds for survival.

Clearly the strategies mentioned here are also effective for individuals who want to try to prevent cancer.

Changing Your Inheritance

"Of all the wonders that I have yet heard,
It seems to me most strange that men should fear,
Seeing that death, a necessary end,
Will come when it come."
William Shakespeare, Julius Caesar

Belief around the time of Shakespeare was that the time of our death is determined by fate. Today we know that we can postpone the date that medicine predicts for us.

Here is an example of negative stress resulting from memories and mindset.

Susan did not have cancer but she told everyone that the women in her family all died of cancer in their fifties and she would too. Nobody had told her she would, she "knew" because her mother, grandmother and their siblings all had. She was really surprised when she turned sixty and was still alive.

This is quite a commonly held belief that can become a self fulfilling prophecy if allowed to persist. Just because your grandparent died of cancer at age 54, doesn't mean you will die at age 54.

First, since your ancestor died there have been huge advances in knowledge, detection and in the treatment of most cancers. Some cancers are now curable, others have become chronic diseases, some are still waiting for a cure.

Secondly, while the genes you inherited may have a propensity to trigger cancer, you may be able to reduce the likelihood of the trigger happening at age 54 by lifestyle choices, stress reduction strategies and the use of cancer fighting agents. Working hard at the suggestions in this book will help you to beat the odds.

Stress From Terror

From those we spoke with, from a psychological sense, people with serious cancer diagnoses, and their loved ones are often initially terrified. They likened this fear to post traumatic stress syndrome.

This terror is partially a hangover from several decades ago when the diagnosis of cancer inevitably meant death. Today the panic is not always as justified because some forms of cancer are now more easily treated and cured. For many though it is still a very scary unknown world .

The main cause of terror is uncertainty and the fear of the unknown. Will I be able to work again? Will I be able to afford all the treatments recommended? How long will I live? How will my family be affected? Are we strong enough to get through this?

Try to be as honest with yourself as you can be. Write down your fears in your journal. Writing them down is a huge part of the process of getting rid of them. Talk them over with your family and trusted team members. If they are really bothering you ask for a referral to a health professional who specializes in helping to reduce psychological stress. The stigma associated with such referrals is now almost zero. There are a few die-hards who still act as if seeing a mental health professional is a sign of weakness. This is left over from wars long ago where individuals with post traumatic stress disorder were shot as cowards. Times have thankfully changed, science has explained the effects of stress, nobody is immune, there is no reason not to ask for help.

Bottled Up Stress

"His wife Jenna told me after he died that although I was helpful and extended his life, he believed so much in what his doctor said that he never really believed anything that I told him. He believed he was going to die, that was what he was told and he did. A psychologist may have been helpful. In my mind he died well before he should have done."

The mind is a powerful thing, our friend or our enemy.

" Eve could not be helped in the least. A friend and excellent reiki healer brought me in two weeks before Eve died. Doctors had sent her home to die. Her breast cancer had returned and metastasized. She had been told that she had months to live, she died earlier than predicted. She was so convinced that she was going to die and had been since her original diagnosis. Our efforts merely reduced the level of pain. Was this an inevitable event or a self fulfilling prophecy? "

The main issue is allowing the fears to multiply in our mind by bottling them inside. We need to get them out in the open. Discussing our issues with someone we respect is key, once it is out in the open it has much less power over us.

The individual diagnosed with cancer has heightened senses, stress does that. They are very sensitive to suggestion. Here is an example; if someone in a position of power, such as a health professional, says "You shouldn't worry, most people with that diagnosis have a couple of years to live, anyway, you might be run over by a bus before then". That statement in itself can be a death sentence. The patient internalizes, "my God, my doctor thinks I have two years at the most".

If however the person in power says, "this is not necessarily a death sentence, the technology is improving, we have treatments and some lifestyle changes we believe you should make", your attitude to the disease would be very different, much more upbeat. Just because past statistics indicate a two year average doesn't mean you will be that average patient or that you cannot change your lifestyle and beat the odds.

David was at the doctors with his wife and daughter. Their hearts stopped when David turned to the doctor and said " well, how long do I have?" They didn't like the answer.

It was interesting, both the daughter and wife independently told me this story; it had clearly affected them deeply. To this day they don't believe that he should have asked the question. More importantly they did not believe that the health professional should have answered in the way he did.

The death "prediction" for many individuals can be like a black magic curse. It doesn't need to be. A psychologist/ spiritual advisor can help you to dig deep and help you see the truth, freeing yourself from such "curses".

In Jane's case the advisor revealed forgotten memories from her childhood that were causing her to have a negative attitude and making her believe that the relatively mild cancer she had was going to kill her.

The memories surrounded the death of her grandmother who everyone told her she was very much like in looks and mannerisms. Jane had subconsciously identified with her grandmother and since she was approaching the age when the grandmother died; she was subconsciously expecting her own death to happen. The psychologist helped her through this and she is alive and well today. Jane admitted she could not have figured this out without an advisors help.

Depression And Stress

Depression is a clinical term, the World Health Organization defines it:

"Depression is a common mental disorder that presents with depressed mood, loss of interest or

pleasure, feelings of guilt or low self-worth, disturbed sleep or appetite, low energy, and poor concentration."

Most normal people have brief periods of depression, it becomes a problem when it is frequent, chronic or very severe.

Most people who have been diagnosed with cancer feel sad, angry, annoyed. Depending on the nature of the diagnosis, how well the health team has delivered the news, what kind of personal resilience and support we have, it can also result in depression.

Treating depression is important, but determining whether you are truly depressed or whether you are experiencing side effects of the treatment (e.g. drug therapy) is often difficult. Sometimes changing the drugs that are prescribed can make the symptoms of depression go away. Depression is a known and sometimes documented side effect of drugs.

Scholarly studies tell us that from 15-30 percent of people diagnosed with cancer are clinically depressed for a time. In my experience with cancer patients, many are depressed initially and few are treated for it. That may not be such a bad thing, often mild depression is a wake up call. Major depression needs professional help immediately.

Don't ignore what your body and mind is telling you. You need to get professional advice however, this is where drugs for depression are sometimes a hindrance. Drugs may mask the symptoms and do not always help the depressed individual to face up to the change in attitude necessary to reduce the long term stress that results from inner conflict. Counseling may be a better option. Sometimes a combination of drugs and counseling is best. Talk to your team, see what is best for you.

Reducing ones inner conflict will reduce the overall stress level and will contribute to improving longevity.

David the Pastor again....." I believe that there are a number of psychological issues that aren't being explored, realize that we are all mortal. Whether this buys you a little time or a lot; whether our coil unwinds now or later, in a car accident or from some other ailment, this event will bring you closer to the wonderful fragility of life, an awareness that makes the value of this gift much closer to our daily living."

David's last point is very important. If we heed Hippocrates advice and look at what we can learn from our illness in all the ways it expresses itself we will emerge stronger and more resilient.

Our friend Deb volunteers at a hospice and counsels dying patients. She tells us it is the most rewarding thing she has ever done. Dealing with death, especially your own is a wonderful thing, if you have the right guide. As the quote from Julius Caesar says, it is something we will all eventually face. Don't leave it until the end, work on it now. A good attitude towards death creates a positive mindset now. It may help you reduce your stress and put cancer more on the back burner.

"Jeff told us his story. The trap I had fallen into was that as I meditated I relaxed and my capacity for stress increased, so I took on more tasks. I was running a business on several continents, paying a mortgage on a house and cottage and trying to be a good father and husband. My life was hectic enjoyable, but manageable. I had become an adrenaline junky, always going for more action, more work, more responsibility.

Disaster struck, it is always the unexpected that throws you the curve, life is not predictable. Surprise! a business partner had left me on the hook for debt he incurred on a project.

Six years of legal hassles later, my retirement money gone, my stress levels were in the stratosphere. My lawyers had proven that my former partner misrepresented the facts and should have been responsible for the debts incurred. Second surprise, *my former partner then declared bankruptcy leaving me to deal with the whole mess.*

My stress levels started to get dangerously close to overload. Anger and frustration started breaking out as I struggled to regain control. A month later, my cancer diagnosis. We cannot predict times like this.

We started trying to reduce the stress load, but that wasn't easy, businesses, house, cottage, mortgages, lines of credit, lawyers fees and vehicles don't disappear overnight. Try as we might we couldn't reduce the stress load fast enough.

We sold our business for what it owed, we sold the house in the city paid down the debt. Following the radiation therapy we moved to a rural area where I could rest, meditate and avoid people for a while while I regrouped and mellowed out. It was a huge financial regression, but we had eliminated much of the debt that had been a major contributor to our stress.

It is interesting that we put pressure on ourselves to live a certain lifestyle. We try to meet others expectations of us and succumb to the peer and family pressure to perform. Society often judges us by what we own, the house, the area, the technological toys we have, the new drapes, the clothes, the restaurants we eat in, the company we keep.

When we ask the key question, **what is more important our lifestyle or our health**, the latter will always be the answer for the sane person. The problem is that we become trapped in our own tracks, unable to see how we live and how we are damaging ourselves.

How many of you need to ask yourself is my lifestyle contributing to my illness?

To Be Or Not To Be?

As mentioned, from 15 to 30 percent of cancer patients are diagnosed as being clinically depressed. Most of the remainder are depressed sometimes. This is often due to the recurrence of the cancer, the experience of regular pain, the quality of life being negatively affected; or due to secondary effects such as loss of employment, underlying drug and alcohol dependency, homelessness, lack of support from friends and family, etc.

Clearly, if you already have major unresolved issues or a past history of trauma or post traumatic stress disorder you may need professional help. It is often in people who don't think they have a problem that issues are hardest to resolve. You have met them, they are out there, they don't listen to reason and they probably won't read this book.

In an earlier book "Meditation for Enduring Happiness" there is a chapter on stress and its effects on brain chemistry. The whole book is about becoming happier and reducing sadness in your life. Here are some key research findings;

1. You can change your brain!
2. You can change the way you react to situations and people.
3. Happiness may not be what you have experienced for most of your life, but it is something you can develop.
4. Becoming happy, having enduring happiness is achievable by everyone, without drugs or alcohol. You can do it yourself by following certain steps outlined in the book.
5. Let me repeat, contrary to popular opinion, research has shown we can change, we can become more happy.

Transforming Yourself

"Courage and cheerfulness will not only carry you over the rough places in life, but will enable you to bring comfort and help to the weak-hearted and will console you in the sad hours"

Sir William Osler

Cancer patients (for that matter patients in general) get caught up in the physical aspects of their disease for two reasons. First, the medical staff tend to stick to the physical symptoms since that is what they know best. Second, patients and health professionals are poorly trained and / or knowledgeable of mind based issues so they don't address them.

This is an issue since several studies have found that cancer patients who work hard at transforming their psychological attitudes live three times longer than those who don't. Thinking positively has been shown to significantly help recovery and longevity.

"***Cancer patients who work hard at transforming their psychological attitudes live three times longer than those who don't***!"

This is an amazing finding. It is proof that mind over matter is a very real concept. Neuro-plasticity research has revealed that we can literally change the structure of our brains/ minds. We can reduce the number of negative thoughts we have, we can become more positive. Every patient with cancer would benefit from working on being more positive.

This is how it works, when we reduce our negative thought patterns the brain structure changes, stress chemicals aren't released, "good" chemicals are released, then it is easier to remain positive and happy. The chronic exposure to the chemicals released due to negative stress contributes to immune system degradation as well as adding stress to your overall stress load. Science has shown that reducing this negative stress translates into increased longevity and beating the odds with cancer.

Dealing With Stress

If your concerns are severe or intense you will need to see a professional.

If they are mild, meditate on your list of fears. Try to remove yourself from the fear and look at it. This is the technique of viewing the self, part of the practice of mindfulness. Look at reactions, feelings, negative thought patterns don't judge, simply try to document it all. Simply bringing it into the light gently helps it dissolve. Remember not to judge the thoughts or allow them to disturb you. Look at the thought as an interesting thing, a mere thing the mind does. Using meditation techniques like this that help you monitor the way your mind works will help you to find out what is behind that fear.

Is it the fact that a close friend or relative died of cancer? Is it something the doctors said? Is it a genetic history? Dig into your past, remember the conversations that may have influenced your feelings about cancer, meditate on them and change that dialog in your head to a positive one. Visualize yourself successfully dealing with the fear. Reread the unifying theory in the appendix and feel empowered in your ability to modify your lifestyle and beat the odds.

Thoughts aren't bad, recurring negative thoughts are unhelpful, take the time to learn how to reconfigure your brain to be happy.

Reflect without judgement on what your underlying feelings are, take your time, sit, be quiet, close the eyes or keep them slightly open. Just reflect on your situation. Make a list, separate your list into different columns; those associated with progression of the disease, those about your upcoming treatment, and others of a personal nature. We can be happy in the midst of a crisis if we find the inner peace that is within us all.

Ask your self these questions:

Is the team of people you have assembled capable of assisting you with your concerns and answering these questions? Just because someone is a great health professional doesn't mean they are good counsellors. Good counseling takes skill and experience, often psychologists, priests, pastors, spiritual guides are better counsellors.

Men in particular often have difficulty discussing issues of a personal nature. Who can you discuss such issues with? Joking with the boys may be pleasant but it doesn't get to those raw issues, find someone you can really talk with.

Are you afraid of asking some team members certain questions, so, do you need to decide which team members you ask which questions? Remember, it is your team, your life, don't be afraid to ask for help. There are many people out there who only need to be asked. Contact your local cancer society for information about volunteer individuals with special skills who may help you.

With respect, the answer to the question: "Do you need a psychologist?"should always be yes! As mentioned, some individuals seem to consider seeing a psychologist as a sign of weakness. My advice is to get over that. Simply put, the observer sees more of the game. A psychologist or advisor will provide insights that you will not see. At this point in your disease progression a spiritual or psychological coach will be very helpful. Seeing an advisor is a sign of strength, not weakness. Going out for a round of golf is nice, relaxing, therapeutic even, but it won't get at those deeper psychological issues.

Years ago I had to see a psychologist to overcome communication issues when presenting to large groups of people. My psychologist Brian helped me to solve my issue in a few sessions. My only wish is that I had seen him earlier, he was an enormous help and continues to be a great friend. Nobody needs to know you have seen a "shrink", and the added benefit is that the psychologist, psychiatrist or spiritual advisor won't tell any of your friends your innermost secrets.

Detoxifying

One real unexpected benefit of a lifestyle change is that you will successfully eliminate contact with toxic people, negative people that you had to interact with (rather than chose to interact with). Toxic relationships cause stress, try to eliminate these relationships! Later, when you are feeling stronger and able to deal with the issues they raise you may decide to allow them back in your life.

This is especially important for individuals who spend all their life as “fixers”; helping others to deal with their problems, they may become drained by the constant stream of demands on their kindness when they are sick. To be of further help to others, you need to take time to look after yourself.

Take Charge Of Your Life

This is your life, only you can change your life. That being said, it does help if your team includes people who are positive and will tell you the truth. Nobody completely understands why some people get cancer and others in the same psychologically toxic environment don’t. Part of it is about being mentally resilient. Resilience can be learned, and improved upon,“Meditation for Enduring Happiness” has information on improving your mental toughness/ resilience.

Getting Away From Toxic People

If you cannot get away physically, get away mentally, find a space, or spaces that are quiet (by the lake or sea is my favourite). Walk the beach, the woods, find a church that is open and empty. Find a room that is quiet. Many hospitals now have quiet rooms or chapels.

Decide to do nothing, just be. Close your eyes, listen to the world around you. Focus on your breath, breathe in, pause, breathe out, pause. Thoughts come, write them in your journal, go back to just being. Breathe in, pause, breathe out, pause. If thoughts come just write them down. Continue, repeat. Notice how your body adjusts to just being.

Body scanning techniques, breathing techniques, techniques that instill quiet and reduce negative thinking are helpful.

Sensitivity To Suggestion

As mentioned earlier, fear due to a cancer diagnosis seems to promote emotional sensitivity. It is hard to avoid if you are diagnosed with cancer and even harder if you are told there is no cure and you are given a timeline that is much shorter than you expected.

Every ache, pain, rash, headache, unusual bowel movement, colour change or feeling is magnified by the mind into a potential problem. This phenomenon has two sides, it is bad if you obsess and good if it triggers you to check out potential problems that could be cut off at the pass before they escalate. This latter path also puts the concern to rest.

"Alex tells of his experience. My experience with a cancer diagnosis is case in point. For several years I ignored symptoms that should have had me going to

the doctor. Doctors didn't offer a PSA test or digital rectal exam and I didn't push for them.

Fortunately, we decided to apply for more life insurance and they insisted on a medical, I failed the medical due to a PSA of 80 (normal is between 0-4). This was followed by a biopsy (which showed Gleason 9) and CT scan, showing lymph gland involvement, the dreaded metastases. Denial and ignoring signals from my body had not been very smart obviously.

Suddenly medical health professionals treated me with kid gloves, I was told I was "palliative" had less than 2 years to live. When your health team treats you like you are the walking dead it is hard not to become a hypochondriac. Every itch, pain, ache, sore spot or muscle spasm could be the cancer becoming more aggressive or starting up again after remission.

Following radiation my blood count was down, and that was expected. After 18 months it was still low. The effects of the radiation should be over by 18 months. One health professional thought it might be an iron deficiency, so that was tested, that wasn't it.

So then the speculation begins, is it the cancer, is the anemia a chronic disease (whatever that is?), or something else. In the midst of these emails back and forth to different members of my health team I had a thought, could this be a side effect of the drugs I was being given. The drug companies site didn't mention it.

Finally, the oncologist wrote back that anemia was a documented side effect of the drug. This was a relief. Most likely the anemia was a side effect and it wasn't the return of the dreaded cancer."

This type of mini drama is played out every day in the lives of people diagnosed with cancer. How patients handle the mini drama is dependent on our ability to deal with stress. How resilient are we to negative stress, do we panic, do we obsess, do we become depressed or do we deny we have an issue? Learn to lead your mind to a place that deals with the facts non-judgmentally. This will help you to find peace.

More On Stress

Let me clear that up; not moron stress, more on stress! Almost everyone has a hard time determining how much stress they have at any particular point in time. Humans are good at many things but determining how much stress they are under and how it is affecting them is not one of them.

Stress is cumulative, each minor stress can add on to existing minor stress and if enough are added we have medium stress, then major stress. If you have minor stress and you get a major one it could put you over the top. If you have a lot of minor stresses, then we add one more, that can put you over the top. The proverbial straw that broke the camels back.

We all have our limits, just look at those brave individuals who go into battle and end up with PTSD, they know what over the top stress is. One source claims that one in five US soldiers returning from Iraq/ Afghanistan has post traumatic stress disorder.

This means that those individuals are at risk of compromised immune systems. Epidemiologists will undoubtedly document an increase in many diseases, including depression and cancers in that group due to the PTSD if left untreated.

Anyone can suffer from too much stress, many great people have suffered including stalwarts throughout history like Sir Winston Churchill, Sir Isaac Newton, Beethoven,

Abraham Lincoln, Hemingway, Tolstoy, the list is endless. It is not weakness, it is overload. The point is that even very famous and notably brilliant minds sometimes misjudge their stress levels and suffer as a result of a sudden event or cumulative smaller events. So don't think you are a bad judge of your self, realize it is a normal human condition and either learn to deal with it, get help or both.

During my battle with "over the top" stress my wife pointed out to me that what I was experiencing was "normal" given the circumstances, and I needed to meditate a little more, cut off my appointments, exercise, eat properly and just relax. It worked, but I am not sure I could have come to that realization myself at the time.

Try this approach, protect yourself by refusing appointments that you know may be stressful. Establish a strong buffer between your current stress load and your limit, then double it. Take a nap every afternoon and listen more closely to what your family and friends say about your stress level.

The cancer treatments may make you weaker and you may need to reduce stress levels even more. There may be no way you can return to your previous stressful job or profession, accept that. Sometimes we cannot conceive of lifestyle changes, you may need to rethink your entire life.

My advice to you is simple, set aside your ego and your pride. Ask your family and trusted friends to assess your stress level, get them to evaluate;

- Are you acting differently?
- Have you had minor falls, car accidents, dropping dishes lately?
- Is your temper close to the surface?
- Have you “lost it” recently?
- Are you less engaged with life?
- Are you watching more TV?
- Are you exercising less?
- Are you drinking too much alcohol, taking drugs, or gambling?
- Are you less happy?
- Is your patience wearing thin?

If some of the answers are yes then ask for a referral to a psychologist or individual or group that can help. In the cancer treatment arena there are many groups that can provide valuable support. There are cancer survivors who are willing to spend time with you.

As the guru says, “change is not just in your pocket, change comes from within” creating change is difficult. In my experience it requires 110 percent of your concentrated effort. It requires you to involve your entire health team, family and friends. It is worth the effort.

CHAPTER NINE - Hope And Beyond Hope

"Nothing in life is more wonderful than faith – the one great moving force which we can neither weigh in the balance nor test in the crucible"
Sir William Osler

Hope is not necessarily a religious concept, atheists can have hope too. That being said, this chapter is not religious as such but touches on some areas that have been the main domain of religion in the past.

Here is a classic story from the eastern meditative traditions:

An older woman came to see a spiritual master. She came into the room, and sat in front of the master, and emotionally said: " My doctor has given me only a few months to live. I am dying, please help me."

In a gentle yet compassionate way, the master began to chuckle, then said: " We are all dying. It's only a matter of time. Some of us just die sooner than others."

As the story goes, the master goes on to help her to see the universality of death. She comes to understand that her impending death is not unique. This reduces her stress. Then the master talks to her about her death and accepting death.

The master gives her a meditation healing practice that she follows enthusiastically. Not only does she come to accept death, but by following the practice with complete dedication, she recovers her health.

Stories like this are common in Buddhist and Yogic spiritual texts. There are no medically documented cases like this that we could find in the literature, but we stay open minded.

Hope Springs Eternal

"Imagine my surprise when year two came and went and I wasn't dead. Who said God doesn't have a sense of humor. My glass became half full."

Optimists fare better than pessimists when it comes to most things in life and cancer is no exception.

As my friend Mary, an oncologist, says about her health care colleagues:

"If you don't have a positive attitude, if you don't give patients hope, you are in the wrong business." She is right, patients need help staying positive.

If you are positive and your health team is positive you will have a much stronger attitude and be more likely to beat the odds.

So, by now you will be following the advice in this book, exercising, eating well, meditating daily, visioning a healthy body (no, we aren't talking about playboy bunnies or male dancers, we mean your body!). Which brings us to laughing, yes, do it often, get on internet joke lists, watch YouTube funnies, go to comedies, watch funny movies, associate with funny people, try laughing yoga (that concept is sort of funny just thinking about 20 people in a room laughing together). Smiling and laughing is contagious, get your friends and family to work with you to follow the funny side of life.

Become inspired and enthusiastic, read stories about spontaneous remission, miracles, spiritual healing. Much as science has no idea how they work, some do work. The results are well documented.

Talk to people who have survived your type of cancer. My friend Bill was told he would die of cancer 25 years ago, he outlived his doctors! Bill is enthusiastic about the miracle that God performed to keep him well. Bill believes the prayers of his wife and friends worked. He didn't suspect that a miracle happened, he knows it to the core of his being.

How is your mental toughness, are you like Bill?

" June is a fighter. Small and feisty, she approaches her doctors with a million questions and is like a dog with a bone until she gets answers. A voracious reader and internet user she drives her health professionals crazy, but in a nice way. June has a big team, health professionals, friends of friends with similar diagnoses, alternative healers, a friend who is a dietician. June is definitely beating the odds. Most of all, June is happy, really happy and comfortable in her own skin. June treats her illness as a full time job, attending workshops, classes, discussing with friends on the phone and by email and other social media. June is a model for beating the odds."

If you are having difficulty staying hopeful, talk to your team. You may be clinically depressed. Could it be a side effect? You may need to see a health professional, and if the non-drug alternatives aren't keeping you hopeful and positive, you may need drugs that can help. This is not the time to be stoic about your needs. Read chapter eight.

My friend Martin tells this story;" My mum was diagnosed with bladder cancer at the age of 55 - this was in 1969, so thoughts were different then.

Anyway, it was insisted that we were all to pretend that she would survive and recover, even after 2 1/2 years, when she became disabled and it was obvious that she was terminal. Right to the end ,another 6 months we kept up the act. You can imagine the strained atmosphere of visits, with the elephant rampaging about the room. This dishonesty discouraged such visits, which made me feel guilty. The net result was that I, at least, never said a proper goodbye - nor did she - and we were all isolated when we most needed to be together. I would not recommend this approach to anyone."

Being open and honest with yourself and others about your diagnosis is the best course. Obviously you need to be tactful with children and those who are emotional but hiding the truth never works in the long run. Most experts agree that telling patients the truth is best. Perhaps not as bluntly as “do you want to bother with treatment” just caring, compassionately honest, emphasizing the cases that have survived.

Uplifting

Hope is something that lifts us up, makes us smile, makes us laugh and we give others hope by having a positive attitude, even in the midst of news that you would prefer you didn’t hear.

Religious and spiritual people will gain hope from recognizing that rebirth or heaven is not a bad thing. Whatever your belief, it is clear that compassion and wisdom combine to provide us with the capability of helping others, giving them hope in turn gives us hope. We can help those we love by being open and honest about our feelings and about our death.

One piece of advice stuck with me through my treatment process. “You really need to surround yourself with positive people and individuals who are in the business of healing the mind and spirit to balance all the health professionals who are focussed on fixing the body.”

If you can afford it pamper yourself with spa treatments, vacations, time off with loved ones. If not, take the time to be alone, to be artistic, to listen to peaceful music, and to laugh. If you need others to make you happy, find a group of like minded people to share your feelings with, or just to be. Take the time to meditate, pray or just sit and breathe.

"Andrew tells us about his client. William came to me as a skeptic. His wife sent him to get him to relax. He was very uptight about his diagnosis. As a Meditation teacher and Reiki master I knew that some people who came to see me would be helped and many would not. It dismayed me that I couldn't help everyone. William proved to me that even if I couldn't cure everyone, I could still be helpful.

We sat together and talked, we meditated together. Something clicked, he returned, said that he felt better, the pain of his cancer was less. Over a period of a year he came to see me weekly. He told me he was going to die in three months according to his doctor, he had been told to get his affairs in order. William died twelve months later. He only beat the odds by nine months but he came a long way in those months and was thankful for the extra time we bought for him." His wife told me that he died content and with renewed hope.

Healers

Hope is a thing of the spirit, uplifting hope can come from many sources, including healers who raise your spirits through spiritual healing and sometimes heal your body too.

"Elsa never struck me as a religious person. She went to weddings, funerals and baptisms but other than Christmas and Easter never went to a Sunday service. She was diagnosed with breast cancer, the chemo gave her cardiology issues. Her husband whisked her away to Paris with a side trip to Lourdes, the famous spiritual healing place. Her doctors were amazed that her heart had been cured and no trace of cancer was to be found. She confided that western doctors didn't understand so she never told them about her visit."

Not communicating about every treatment you are using to doctors, due to a fear of ridicule, is a common thread through the stories we were told when researching for this book.

Healing has been a major part of many religions for thousands of years, one early documentation is the old testament story of the healing of Naaman by Elisha a Jewish prophet almost three thousand years ago (2 Kings 5: 1-14).

"John tells us about his Nanna. My grandmother was a Christian spiritual healer in the UK in the 1950's and 60's and she often healed me as a child. Aches and pains disappeared with her touch. She never charged for any healing. She said her healing ability came from God and she healed because the energy of God's love flowed through her to the person she was healing."

There are some amazing things in this world that science has yet to explain and the healing intention, healing by touch alone is one of those things. Churches have medical evidence of such miracles, the documentation of such healing has been well publicized.

Suggestion Or Placebo

Medical science tells us it is the placebo effect. Usually explained as "if you give a child a sugar pill and tell them they will be well they often become well". Science often looks down on such healing as "quackery". According to them it is simple minded and foolish. In essence, we cannot explain it so it must be fake, somewhat close minded thinking, hardly what you would expect from a scientist.

The power of suggestion, placebo, or healing touch may be an important medical tool.

"My knee was injured in a car accident. Surgery was apparently going to be needed in the future. A spiritual healer from the spiritualist society laid hands on the injured knee and reduced the pain. That was fifteen years ago, and I have not had surgery yet."

This could easily be explained away as a poor medical diagnosis, or healing related to powerful suggestion by the healer. The person with the injured knee told me, they didn't care, it had worked.

Perhaps this is nothing but the placebo effect. Let us think about this, he has avoided surgery for 15 years, and has lived with a lower perceived level of pain. Perhaps this power of suggestion "trick" is more than that, perhaps it has a very practical application. Perhaps we should do some research.

It is just too easy to write it off as just being "the power of suggestion". There is something very powerful and if harnessed correctly, very healing, going on here.

Almost every health professional with experience will tell you that some people will survive a serious illness because they "have the right attitude". They have more than mere hope, they have a belief that is beyond normal. Physicians who are honest will also tell you that sometimes people defy all odds and are healed by what can only be described as a miracle. They happen, we don't know why.

People who are very positive survive better than individuals with negative attitudes everything else being equal.

To improve your attitude and chances of survival:

- Watch comedies not tragedies,
- Develop a better attitude,
- Read books that inspire,
- Hang out with positive people,
- Do things that make you feel good,
- Help others,
- Love more,
- Pray or meditate, or both
- Take naps,
- Read positive books, spiritual books, comedy,
- Smile, (place a note on your mirror smile),
- Get on a friends email joke list,
- Search out people who make you laugh,
- Sing, to yourself, or better yet, join a choir and sing with others,
- Listen to uplifting music,
- Help with a homeless program, or other volunteer situation,
- Train your mind to be happy using mindfulness meditation .

Document your worries, share them with your team and then let them go. This will help the worries disappear. Often bringing negative thoughts into the light will eliminate them. If that doesn't work, write your worries on a piece of paper and burn it to represent you overcoming the worries.

As a wise woman once said;
Don't worry about the small stuff,
Everything is the small stuff.

Giving your time, enthusiasm and cheerfulness to those in need will give you strength and improve your sense of self worth. Through giving others hope in this way you will build your own hope and love of life. Giving truly is better than receiving. Now you have built back your strength the key next step is giving of yourself to others. You will learn to do this in your way, in your time.

CHAPTER TEN - Enhancing The System

Curing The Whole Person

The World Health Organization definition of health is that :

"Health is a state of complete physical, mental and social well-being and not merely the absence of disease or infirmity."

The medical profession spends most of its time curing the disease and its symptoms, not the whole person. This was as true in Sir William Osler's day as it is today.

This is not a criticism of individual medical practitioners, time is money and health systems are short of money. There are so many cases to help that there is realistically not enough money to buy the time necessary to deal with all the issues of the whole person. Most of the physicians I know would love to have the time each person really needs. The medical reimbursement systems generally do not reward physicians for time spent with patients, or for successful outcomes of treatment either. That is why ***we need to fully integrate volunteers into the system***, not just as people who show you where to go and make you tea, but we need training programs for volunteers to help them take on roles that would support better patient care; roles that are not funded within the system such as system navigators, and counsellors.

Overprescribing

It is easier for the health system to get physicians to prescribe a pill than to teach a patient how to use a time consuming but equally effective cure. Our health systems are currently not capable of treating the whole person. It is up to you to treat your whole person to the best of your ability, nobody else is going to do it for you!

A colleague of ours recounted this story; "Doreen was elderly and had multiple issues. She told us she was taking five prescriptions and was seeing three physicians. The reason we were concerned was that she had blacked out and fallen. Her family practitioner ordered heart tests, neurological tests, and stroke tests at the families insistence. All were normal for her age. With her permission we spoke with the pharmacist about her falls and asked for a printout of the drugs she was taking and their side effects.

The pharmacist chirped in that only one of the drugs she was taking might lead to falls but she shouldn't really be having a problem with any of them. First of all we found two drugs doing the same thing, one ordered by a family doc the other by a specialist. We started to worry. Then we looked up each of the five drugs, two drugs had dizziness as side effects, one caused fainting, so much for the advice from the pharmacist.

The upshot was that in discussions with her doctors the drug was changed, one was dropped all together. The outcome was that the falling stopped. This is an all too common situation, often with drastic results. She could easily have died from this problem.

This is another situation where ***volunteers could be trained to review whether cancer patients and the elderly generally are having issues that may be drug side effect related***. Potential issues could then be brought to the health professionals attention for action.

There is an obvious win-win for electronic health systems that monitor drugs prescribed to detect conflicts and dangerous side effects. Such systems are in the process of being implemented in most organized health systems in the world. These systems will improve care for patients and pay for themselves by preventing drug interactions.

Indignity

They say that the first thing lost in war is the truth, well the first in healthcare is dignity. Not the obvious indignities such as squeezing your breast on to a mammography machine, or having a digital rectal exam. Such activities are necessary.

No, the indignity that we heard about from cancer patients was the flippancy of some professionals who treated them without care or respect. While keeping a psychological distance with critically ill patients is one of the defense mechanisms it is not how patients should be treated.

In addition there is the indignity of being ignored, made to wait long periods of time for no apparent reason and generally being treated with arrogance by some health professionals.

To summarize, while most health professionals are excellent, ***some health professionals need to be more positive***, and treat patients as equals, as friends. As my friend Mary says about her fellow cancer professionals, if they can't be positive and give hope, they are in the wrong business.

System Cracks

Emily was surprised to learn she had advanced breast cancer at age 80 because for years she and her husband had been paying for private health coverage. What they had failed to tell Emily was that people in the private sector of healthcare in the UK do not automatically get National Health Service notifications to get regular mammograms. Her private health coverage provided her with excellent care for her diabetes, but she fell between the cracks when it came to regular screening. Emily received good care from the specialists she was referred to for her breast cancer treatment. She was told she was lucky, they barely caught the cancer in time.

Cracks exist in every system, so it is really important to take personal responsibility so nothing is missed. The handoff between family physicians and specialists is a common area for problems to occur. Don't assume that your doctor is covering all the areas that need attention.

Professional Arrogance

As a patient and graduate of a program delivered by a Faculty of Medicine I can confirm that the arrogance one experiences from health professionals is taught in University. Our early lectures included descriptions of who we were supposed to be, the "cream that rises to the top"; "you will graduate and immediately have to take charge".

At first you laugh inside your head at the ridiculous ego of it all but after a while it becomes a repeated cliche that you either turn off or begin to believe. The problem with this conditioning is that many health professionals actually begin to believe they have a right to be arrogant.

The consequence is that they think their time is more important than yours, they should have priority parking, drug companies should pay for their $200 per bottle wine at dinner. Perhaps worst, some actually believe that they know best, even though they haven't stayed current.

The professions need to monitor this and start to deal with the arrogant ones.

Improving Data Collection

"George, a good friend who died of cancer worked for years in the weed control industry. When it was revealed that some of the chemicals he had been

breathing in for 15 years were toxic and masks should have been worn, he changed careers and started driving for a delivery service. When he developed lung and brain cancer and was asked his occupation he said driver. Even though his family kept mentioning his 15 years of chemical exposure, there was no line on the form for past employment history so the information wasn't recorded. They tell me this happens every day and a huge opportunity is lost to learn from these tragic cases."

Clearly ***we need to be more diligent about the information we collect about people who have a cancer diagnosis***. Data is now very inexpensive to store, the major problem has been that we don't document all of the relevant data. Data tends to be collected for financial and billing reasons rather than clinical or epidemiological ones.

The focus in health care is on treating the individual with drugs, it should also be on understanding and preventing disease. Collecting and analyzing data is key to making this happen. The author knows from personal and professional experience that in healthcare,once the evidence is there and published, change inevitably happens. Politicians will act if the information is beyond reproach. We also know that, to quote a deputy minister in a health ministry; "sometimes it is better that we don't open that can of worms". Politicians are risk averse, issues may alter the political landscape, so cans of worms are avoided, sometimes to the detriment of patients.

The solution here is to set up an agency with the freedom to focus on information gathering without reporting directly to politicians.

Old Boys (And Now Girls) Network

Several years ago I had the opportunity to interview Sir Ian Kennedy who had headed an inquiry into the deaths of children at an esteemed UK hospital. We have him on tape saying that there was an "old boys culture" which had prevented the real story from coming out sooner. This old boys culture unfortunately protected bad medical practices and bad research among expert physicians. As a result of his work the UK has gone a long way to deal with such issues.

Other jurisdictions still need to work on cutting through the "old boys culture".

Clearly involving bold individuals like Sir Ian, who are not health care professionals and do not have ties to the profession being investigated is key to breaking through the negative effects of the old boys culture.

Education

Education is a life long passion, at least it should be. My former business required me to fly to smaller centres that had hospitals. Often these centers had airports but no commercial flights to their location. Time was valuable so learning to fly small planes to get to meetings and back to my office in reasonable time was cost effective.

The main thing relevant to this discussion that this adventure taught me was that if you wanted to be a pilot you had to be prepared to take many courses and many tests.

Re-testing was mandatory every couple of years and it was more frequent if you were older or flying commercial planes, Pilots are required by law to be current. The result is that the skies are very safe.

***Healthcare could learn a great deal from aviation safety standards*.**

Contrast this with the doctor, who graduated bottom of their class from the worst of the worlds 2,200 medical schools! In many jurisdictions they don't have to re-certify, take courses or be retested. This is true even if they have practiced for 50 years, haven't read any updating service or even opened an article on healthcare.

While the health profession generally encourages professionals to take courses and good health systems require their physicians to take courses to maintain their privileges, in some jurisdictions, unfortunately, they don't have to.

The issue is that this requirement to update their knowledge is not standard across a country or around the world, it is often region specific.

Fortunately, most health professionals **do** choose to take courses and tests regularly, but in many jurisdictions there are no requirements to do so. This is just not logical.

Education and some level of retesting should be mandatory.

Scorecard

How do you know whether a health professional is current? How do you know whether a hospital has a high infection rate? How do you know whether your treatment is state of the art?

Have you ever tried asking a pilot when they were last tested? They will pull out their logbook and answer you without any hesitation; it is so much a part of their profession that they don't think twice. They are in no way insulted by the request, it is part of their culture. They are proud to show you their hours, the planes they have flown, the number of landings made, and the last time they were tested.

Now, try asking a health professional the same question, see their reaction. They act insulted, or think you are joking or they accuse you of making a snide comment about their abilities. The focus of the culture is protection of the individual professional rather than protection of the patient.

The medical culture can be self serving and will close ranks when threatened. As mentioned, Sir Ian Kennedy found this in the UK when he investigated the pediatric deaths in Bristol.

In many jurisdictions it is now common for the performance of professionals to be made available to the public. Surgical rates of infections, mortality rates and other performance related statistics are posted on the internet. Now to be honest, this information can be somewhat misleading. Some excellent regional hospitals take on the most difficult patients that other smaller centers won't touch so their mortality rate is often higher. The numbers can hide the truth somewhat, but for those centers that are good at their work and in demand anyway, publishing the numbers won't affect them.

As the ultimate payor in the system, ***the taxpayer deserves to see what she/he is getting for their money***.

"One study of gynecologists we undertook showed that technique was a major factor that affected the number of their patients that had to return to the operating room because of adhesions. Adhesions occur in some patients following surgery, our study showed that where the surgeon was trained was

often linked to how many of their patients returned for adhesion removal surgery. It depended on the technique they had been taught. The rate of adhesions varied from 3% to over 20%. You will want the gynecologist who had the 3% adhesion rate."

Publishing that kind of information would be helpful.

It would also give physicians the feedback they need to decide if it was time to go back for re-education. Surgeons often don't know what best practice is because until recently the data wasn't collected or shared beyond their own clinical department (if that). In many jurisdictions performance comparison through outcome measurement is just starting to be made available through agencies like NICE in the UK and the Canadian Institute for Health Information. It is hoped that sharing of these performance statistics will enhance continuing education in the medical field.

Volume

"Another reason for the variation in rates of gynecological adhesions was the number of cases they handled each year. The more cases a physician treated the better their performance was with regard to adhesions. This makes sense, it is usual that if

we treat more cases we become more skillful because each case is slightly different and if you have completed a larger volume you are more likely to have seen all the variations before."

Do you know where your doctor was trained, how many cases a year your doctor handles, what his or her success rate is and what the hospital infection rate is? Probably not, but clearly ***we need to encourage government to provide the ultimate payers (taxpayers) with such information***.

Collaboration

Legal liability is a huge part of medicine in the US, elsewhere it is less litigious but specialists have their reputations to think of, being safe is good for the reputation. As a result they tend to stay to their unique specialty.

The result is that health care has become a sea of silo's. Each tower of information is excellent, but limited by the fact it knows little or nothing about the other silo's.

My friend, a very senior and very good oncologist has a pat answer when asked about areas outside his expertize:

"I have no information to support or deny the claim that the approach is effective".

His response is sensible and he believes, in his patients best interests.

The issue with including a naturopathic technique in his treatment recommendations, for example, is that he is afraid he would be going beyond "medicine" and thus he could be legally liable.

When it comes to naturopathy, he hasn't taken the time to research the matter and prefers it that way. Nobody likes to be sued. He can't be sued if he stays safely within the limits of "established" medical practice. The question this poses, is the threat of legal liability limiting good patient care and potentially causing patients damage or even death?

As mentioned in chapter one, the volume of health articles is now so large that the average specialist reads only articles from their specialty. Agencies that provide them with reviews of articles for a price have to limit the breadth of the review. Reviewers are expensive. So specialists review only those articles directly related to their area of expertise that are listed in top tier journals. So, they have no idea that naturopaths are effective, in addition their patients don't tell them and their peers would criticize them. In my view patient care is being compromised by this approach.

System funding agencies need to create financial models that research and support collaboration.

This narrow approach of working only with medical practitioners reduces the specialists risk of being sued for malpractice. That is another reason why the commercial update houses are so popular. There can be no criticism or threats of law suits for medical negligence if they stay within the knowledge base that is shared by and agreed to by their peers.

The people we interviewed felt the systems would be more effective if teams included medical and alternative team members.

Today, we have some group practices, Family Health Teams, HMO's, CHC's and other groupings that have emerged over the last few decades where groups of healthcare professional work together to provide patient care. Even though these agencies have brought nurses and physicians together within the same organization there are still some health team members not available in these settings leaving care gaps for those with a cancer diagnosis.

As mentioned, many cancer patients need the support of psychologists, social workers and alternative health providers. One recent study found that 80 percent of cancer patients used alternative therapies. Lets think about that for a moment, four out of five patients are using two different systems of care. Each system is convinced that the other is flawed.

My Oncologist laughs at any mention of alternative therapies so I don't mention it. My Naturopath throws up her hands at the apparent lack of testing for things like allergies that could contribute to cancer treatment and the medical systems lack of concern about drug side effects. Who loses in this situation; the patient and the health system.

Patients have to deal with the fact that they are piggy in the middle. The patients we interviewed didn't know if the medical people or the alternative ones were right.

We all know of individuals who have said they will only listen to their medical doctor, or only to their alternative therapy person. Were they right?

That being said there are recent research papers that reveal a combination of alternative and allopathic medicine is the best path to follow.

More research on this would be appropriate if it were followed up by action. We all need to push our politicians and health care providers for action to improve health care collaboration.

Cure The Whole Patient

Medicine has evolved into a practice that attempts to cure symptoms of disease not the whole patient. Sir William Osler commented on this a century ago and it is still a problem today. One reason alternative practitioners are so popular is that they often look at the whole patient. Health information is so voluminous that we can no longer expect individual practitioners to understand all there is to be known in order to work on the whole patient. We need health teams that work together for the good of the patient. Expecting individual practitioners to volunteer to give up control is expecting too much.

Government intervention is needed to create large comprehensive health teams and phase out the silo's.

Medical Industrial Complex

We have had a great experiment for the last fifty or more years. Drug companies have been naively trusted to do what is best for patients; they have proven that first they will do what is best for their corporation.

Sometimes the "System" develops a momentum in one direction while other equally brilliant minds show that the direction is not the optimal one. Often the direction that wins out is the one that lines the pockets of major corporations.

In health care, products can be patented if they meet certain criteria. This is good, research is expensive and individuals and corporations need to be able to recover what they invested to develop a treatment. With a patent you are protected from competition, so if you market well you can be guaranteed to make returns on your investment.

If on the other hand your product is effective but cannot be patented, all your research efforts go unpaid. Corporations need revenue to survive, so with some minor exceptions only "patentable" products are pursued through research, this isn't a conspiracy, just a fact. The problem is that this no patent, no profit, no research policy has resulted in huge increases in drug costs in healthcare with potentially low cost alternatives not being researched or implemented.

Government funding should be made available for research. Not only will it potentially have significant cost benefits to society but it may save many lives. If curcumin, melatonin, IV vitamin C and green tea extract, for example, actually do prove to be effective cancer treatments using "gold standard research", the savings to the health systems around the world could be huge.

Drug companies are not going to do this research. If they find green tea extract effective for example, they will either bury the research and come out with another product, or try to patent a unique "drug" that is actually the active ingredient of green tea using another name. They would then sell it for thousands of dollars per patient further bankrupting the health system.

If on the other hand the government found green tea extract effective, everyone would benefit from the low cost solution.

We cannot afford to continue to abdicate healthcare research strategy to the drug companies by allowing them to set the research agenda.

As health budgets continue to be constrained any effective solution that is less expensive than drugs needs to be seriously considered. Financial savings that would potentially result would free up resources to help with more research and better treatment. Such research is imperative until a cure for cancer and other diseases are developed.

A major problem for those of us diagnosed with cancer is when effective methods of saving lives are not researched because the product would not be profitable.

So the issue for those diagnosed with cancer is that the lack of gold standard research doesn't necessarily mean that the alternative healthcare product is not effective. Non-patentable solutions are generally less expensive for individuals and the health system, they may also have fewer side effects. Consequently it would be really good if we could evaluate the effectiveness of the non-patentable products.

Approval by the FDA and other regulators would best serve the public if drugs were compared with non patentable alternatives as well as a placebo.

"The No Patent, No Profit, No Research Tax".

Alternatively, since the government issued patent is a privilege not a right, taxpayers, represented by government, have the right to set terms. One of those terms could be ***a tax on gross profits of drug companies to go into a fund to research those items that cannot be patented but show evidence of efficacy.***

Side Effects

Side effects need to be better documented for cancer patients who are faced with treatment decisions. Nobody can make good decisions if the information is weak or missing.

Clinical trials need to supply improved side effect data as part of the condition of getting approval. A database of side effects needs to be documented and raw data made available to researchers for more effective evaluation of drugs versus alternatives. Side effects need to be tracked as do drug interactions and patient outcomes as discussed earlier in this book.

Placebo

Spontaneous remission associated with placebos needs to be documented in clinical trials and the data made available to researchers.

Drug companies need to supply such data as part of the documentation required to get drug approval. The placebo effect needs to be treated as a serious research opportunity and understood from all aspects including spiritual.

Psychology

The psychological effects of a cancer diagnosis need to be considered more carefully. Dealing with depression in cancer patients is imperative to attain more positive outcomes. Reducing the incidence of depression in cancer patients will improve the outcomes of cancer treatment.

Psychologists and counsellors should routinely be made available to cancer patients in need.

Navigation

Cancer patients need system navigators, because the needs of the cancer patient cut across many health care disciplines. Coordination between disciplines is weak or non-existent. ***Patient care navigators who support the patient and ensure cross discipline communication would be a real asset to the care delivery system.***

Stress

The theory in Appendix one relies heavily on the fact that stress is additive whether it is physical stress or psychological stress. Although there are many articles linking stress and cancer, many physicians are not aware of this information.

Information on stress and cancer needs to be distributed to health professionals.

It is another research situation that needs further work. The Unifying theory clearly indicates that reducing stress does assist in beating the odds.

The financial benefit to the health care systems worldwide could be immense if this theory was researched then acted on. Stress can often be relieved through low tech therapies with obvious benefits

The bottom line is that this research work will be done in the fullness of time. Just as the meditation research work was done eventually when the body of information became overwhelming.

In this situation however we could prevent thousands if not millions of premature deaths by doing our due diligence now. Lets not waste any more time.

Be well, be happy.

Michael J.McCartney MES, MHSc.
April 2012.

APPENDIX ONE - Unifying Theory

"The first duty of the physician is to educate, not to prescribe medicine."

Sir William Osler

There is currently no unifying theory of cancer to help patients understand how best to proceed once diagnosed with cancer. In addition a unifying theory would potentially help those who would like to try to postpone or prevent cancer

There are many scholarly discussions about "bits" of a theory, most require a good science background to understand. One example is the current debate about whether metastasis is due to cancer cells acting like white blood cells. Another is the purpose of telomeres. Telomeres are said to limit the life of chromosomes and when they go wrong may lead to cancer. These theories deal with disaggregated pieces of cancer development or metastases and they tend to be physical in nature. The prevailing genetic theories for example give patients the impression that their fate is in the hands of their genes and there is nothing they can do to change that fate. Even genetic experts will tell you that this is not necessarily a linear process that you cannot change. These theories are not helpful to patients who have a form of cancer that has no cure. Clearly they need to be able to understand what they can do.

Here is the usual way that oncologists and cancer researchers and organizations explain cancer to patients and families(source-flyers handed out by cancer centres):

1. *Something goes wrong and one or more mutations alters one or more genes*
2. *In some cases, the altered gene sends a wrong message*
3. *Often, the cell begins to divide rapidly*
4. *The cell forgets to stop dividing.*
5. *It forms a lump or tumour.*

There is a "silent" period when cancer cells are dividing and there are no associated symptoms /health issues, then when a certain number is reached the tumour or its effects on the body are noticeable and a diagnosis occurs.

Screening may identify cancer before symptoms are seen using various markers.

A variation of this basic cancer theory is that we carry "Oncogenes" (cancer genes) along with our normal genes but they aren't activated in a normal body. There is some evidence that certain patients have certain genes and contract certain cancers the problem is that they aren't found in all cases so causality is not proven.

The oncogenes or gene mutation occurs when one or more carcinogens, activates or mutates the cell. Carcinogens are things like smoke, food contaminants, viruses, etc."

Unifying Theory

In the common explanations above, which are paraphrased from a number of sources, there are words like“something happens” or “often”which really means “we don’t know what happens” or worse, it is too complex to explain to a layperson.

The other problem with this way of explaining cancer is that it is too linear. The impression we are left with is that cancer happens and there is nothing you can do about it. It will progress along a path and other than the treatment we recommend there is no way out of this situation.This is not a correct or a helpful way of presenting the information. Individuals diagnosed with cancer need to know this is not an inevitable path.

Clearly as an oncologist friend said to me “Michael, to be honest, we don’t know anything about cancer other than some things seem to work on some people some of the time.”

He was being humble, cancer researchers actually know many things about cancer, but he was right in that there is no consistent unifying theory for cancer. This lack of a macro view of cancer is not helpful to those patients who have to wait for a cure. Our minds need to be sure to make sense of the cancer to feel in control of it, the unifying theory helps.

Here is our synthesis of the large amount of evidence we analyzed in preparing this book, for want of a better name we are calling it the ***Unifying theory of Cancer.***

Hypothesis One:The development of cancer is not a linear process but a circular one.

What we mean by this is that the body is very good at fighting disease. There are many self regulating systems within the body.

The facts show that Cancer has many false starts in the body that are controlled by the bodies self regulating systems before it proliferates to a point where it becomes an issue.

The circularity explains things like spontaneous remission. The cancer starts for some reason, then it slows or stops as the body's environment changes. We know that many cadavers have cancer cells even though that is not what they died from.

More importantly for us, this circularity explains why certain individuals beat the odds and live far beyond their doctors expectations.

What we need to understand is why this happens in some individuals but not in others, why the variability?

Why are some individuals in the same environment with the same exposure to toxins resilient and not others?

Stress

Stress is more than psychological, it is also physical. Pain is an example of physical stress, but so is being chronically tired or overweight or suffering from a chronic disease.

Physical stress and the relationship to cancer has been known for a long time. In 1775 a British surgeon linked chimney soot to a form of cancer unique to chimney sweeps. It wasn't until 1918 that researchers were able to actually induce cancer on the earlobes of rabbits using tar. Carcinogens like tar and soot can trigger cancer in certain individuals. It depends on the levels of the carcinogen and the resilience of the individual to cancer.

Chronic diseases like diabetes are a different example of physical stress. While diabetes is a disease of the pancreas, the liver is also compromised by diabetes (fatty liver formation) and the liver is a critical organ for detoxing the body naturally. Diabetics are more likely to get certain cancers due to the stress of more compromised immune systems and the reduced liver and pancreatic function.

It is well known that psychological stress (pain, depression, etc.) causes chemicals to be released in the body. This is a natural part of the bodies self regulatory process, the problem is not occasional chemical releases in response to daily living but the chronic exposure to these naturally occurring chemicals. It has been found that certain stress related corticosteroids cause the hippocampus in the brain to reduce in size with resultant neural deficits. Some of these chemicals have now been linked to cancer. Adrenaline for example, released in reaction to negative stress has been recently shown to accelerate tumor growth. Psychological stress such as depression or PTSD increases the likelihood of getting cancer. So both physical (body) stress and psychological (mind/brain) stress are implicated in cancer.

Hypothesis Two : Stress from different sources is additive.

Negative thinking causes stress, physical strain causes stress, trauma causes stress and physical disease cause stress. Is it possible that the combined stress causes the body to release chemicals which causes metabolic stress? Does the stress in combination help to overload the bodies self regulating mechanisms and thus trigger cancer cells to proliferate? So is it that individuals who are genetically resilient, or have learned to control stress are less likely to trigger cancer cell proliferation?

Hans Selye the celebrated researcher, found that psychological stress was additive. Changing jobs, having an argument, etc. each adds to the stress load.Minor stresses were shown to add up to become like major stresses.

In the unifying cancer theory we take this one step further. In addition to psychological stress being additive, we theorize that psychological, metabolic, physiological and respiratory stresses are all additive. This is logical.

Here is an example of physical stress being additive. Over sixty years ago it was shown that half of the patients with asbestosis went on to develop lung cancer, but if the patient smoked tobacco, that percentage increased significantly. This started the theory that multiple hits on a gene was more likely to trigger cancer. However there were always anomalies in the data that were ignored. There were individuals who both smoked and were exposed to asbestos but survived. Nobody at the time asked why.

Psychological stress also contributes to cancer, this is well documented in holocaust survivors for example who are known to experience higher rates of cancer than the general population.

It makes sense that all types of stress are also additive. We see this in patients with multiple diseases. As a simple example, if your body is hot, it is a very hot day, your reaction to a minor infection is much worse. Our emergency departments become full in hot weather, respiratory ailments amplify, as do other diseases. So we see the additive nature of stresses every day in healthcare.

As we are exposed to environmental stress, psychological stress, chronic diseases such as asthma, heart disease, diabetes, the stresses add up and contribute to two things; additive stress compromises the immune system response and the bodies ability to repair mutations to the gene sequence is compromised. It is not just genetics.

Researchers tell us that gene mutations occur every day and are repaired every day in a "normal" person. However, we theorize, when advancing age and/or exposure to bacteria or viruses, or toxins in food, water and air add up they cause stress to the body.

In terms of gene mutations, we theorize that with increasing stress, the normal repair mechanisms cannot keep pace with the number of negative mutations and the result is a change either to the gene or its function.

This is not the only effect, combine this with the fact that stress compromises the immune system and we have a double impact. Cells in a particular area of the body start becoming cancerous. Instead of unhealthy cells dying normally, cancer cells proliferate.

The Unifying theory explains why people living in relatively toxin free environments, avoiding foods and drink that contain toxins, live a relatively stress free life and are physically active have lower incidences of cancer. The same people move to a developed country with pollution, daily stress, toxic people and toxic food and water and cancer cell proliferation is triggered at a younger age. It is our pollution, the invisible chemicals in our food, our homes, coming out of our cars and in our air and water that are killing us. Cancer prevention involves cleaning up our planetary mess. It involves growing organic food and learning to treat our own bodies with respect. Seventh day adventists who are vegetarian and don't smoke or drink alcohol fare much better than the individuals they work alongside. This is consistent with the theory.

Hypothesis Three: Cancer cycles according to the total stress load over time.

The proliferation of cancer cells may slow or stop by itself and not proceed. We know this because many autopsies reveal a presence of undiagnosed, cancer unrelated to the cause of death.

In these situations we theorize that either stress was low level and so the cancer was kept relatively under control or that stress peaked and then dropped back to lower levels.

Total stress levels in the body will vary day by day according to exposure levels to carcinogens, psychological stress level variation and other stress. At some point the stress level exceeds the tipping point and cancer proliferation exceeds cancer control. The next day, if levels drop, cancer gene repair, immune system capability and available cancer fighting foods may combine to bring cancer back under control.

This part of the hypothesis is key to beating the odds. If you get diagnosed, immediately start reducing all the negative psychological, physiological and other stress from your life. Individual chapters in this book will help with that.

Hypothesis Four: Current medical treatment may not be enough

There are new designer drugs for some cancers that are very effective, but for most cancers there is only traditional treatment options. Classical medical treatment usually involves one or more of chemical targeting of the cancer, radiation of the cancer or removal of the tumor by surgery. If all the affected cells are removed this may be successful.

The issue is that not all cancer cells may die and the cancer may return. If the treatment did not get all the cancer cells <u>and you continue to live the way you did before the treatment </u>(i.e. with the same stress levels) chances are better that the cancer may return. If you reduce your stress load in addition to having medical treatment you will still be better off and have a better chance of beating the odds.

In addition, the medical industrial complex has created a situation where the drugs approved and the medical culture may not include alternative products and services that are also effective cancer fighting solutions. Unfortunately we must go outside the current medical system to other professionals such as naturopaths and nutritional counsellors to obtain other evidence based help.

Evidence shows that diet, exercise and certain supplements may be very helpful in reducing the liklihood of cancer returning.

Further Evidence

So, based on this theory, to slow the rate of regrowth we would need to reduce our existing stress levels, in every way, physical, psychological and metabolic. In other words eat and live in a healthy manner that we know avoids triggering cancer cell proliferation.

Alternative or complementary supplements will probably be part of the arsenal used to keep cancer growth rates in check.For example, therapies such as green tea extract target cancer cells and cancer blood supply and so may slow cancer growth rates. Also, antioxidants and supplements such as blueberries and cur-cumin have been shown to cause cancer cell death in the lab. Melatonin is also a powerful antioxidant but it also directly affects mitochondria in a positive way as well as gene repair and so may have extra value.

In addition to reducing stress levels, considering food as medicine is a proven way to fight cancer. Eating more cancer fighting foods will be effective according to this unifying theory, foods that are known cancer fighters such as cruciferous vegetables and a vegetarian diet generally. On the other hand foods that are used as fuel by cancer cells such as white sugar contribute to negative body stress and should be avoided in this model of cancer.

Aerobic exercise has been shown to assist with gene repair and to reduce stress by release of "good" stress chemicals, it is cancer fighting.

So, in summary, how do we deal with cancer in a way that helps us to beat the odds?

In essence we need to create an environment that is not cancer conducive and that is free of stress in every sense of the word; psychological, chemical, metabolic and physiological stressors.

Avoiding Negative Theories

Focussing on genes as the only theory isn't healthy. Our preoccupation with a gene-only model dates back to the 1950's and the advances since then in identifying genetic causes of disease. The gene model alone does not explain why some get cancer and others don't since many with cancer don't have the gene markers. The reality has to be more than that simple genetic model which is linear and without hope for those without a cure.

The unifying theory answers many more questions, empowers the cancer patient and through the circularity indicates that we may overcome or significantly slow the cancer through our actions.

Medical research confirms that alcoholics, diabetics, people exposed to carbon monoxide, individuals exposed to certain toxins and individuals under stress all may experience higher than normal acidity in the blood. For this to happen the normal regulatory mechanism has to become disrupted.

Remember in developed countries there are currently more "abnormal" people than "normal" people due to obesity, diabetes, addiction, depression, pollution and stress. Cancer rates are higher, this is not a coincidence. Diabetes affects just under 10 percent of the population in "developed" countries, so called pre-diabetics are another 10 percent. In 2009, 10 percent of Americans were taking antidepressants, that is probably higher now. Seventy percent of the population report more stress now than five years ago, and just about everyone in the west is exposed to more toxins or carcinogens.

Stress Detection

One of the benefits of the Unifying theory is as follows.

In the same way that diabetes may be dealt with easily if detected early, patients may benefit from research into "pre-cancer" patients. Predicting future cancer probability, as with predicting diabetes would provide an opportunity to both intervene and educate the patient about lifestyle changes that may be necessary to slow or eliminate cancer onset.

Intervention Research

These are potential areas for further intervention research for cancer prevention. They are a code to live by.

• Reduce toxins in food. Toxins accumulate in fat, they accumulate even more in animal fat, including ours. If you must eat meat, eat lean meat. Avoid organ meat such as the liver which filters out toxins and can be very high in toxin levels. Vegetables and fruit that are truly organic are less likely to have been blasted by pesticides and will expose an individual to less toxins.

• Wash pesticides off with a vinegar and baking soda solution or soap and water.

• Avoid cancer promoting foods, avoid simple sugars, sweets, candy and alcohol. These items are cancer fuel.

• Reduce weight sensibly. This not only reduces stress on the liver but also boosts the immune system.

• Consider talking with a naturopath about taking Melatonin each night to help regulate sleep, act as an antioxidant improve gene repair and protect normal cellular mitochondria.

• Consider consuming antioxidants such as green tea extract, blueberries and cur-cumin to promote apoptosis (death) of cancer cells.

• Exercise every day, both Yoga type exercise and aerobic exercise. Yoga to improve flexibility, improve blood flow, lymph system flow and generally improve breathing, and aerobic exercise such as fast walking, jogging to help keep weight in balance, help gene repair and improve heart health.

• Learn to breathe deeply, try pranayama or yogic breathing. The Nobel Prize in 1931 went to Warburg who showed that cancer was caused by a lack of oxygen at the cellular level. Breathing properly helps oxygenate the blood so that oxygen is available at the cellular level. Yogi's practice this deep breathing pranayama daily and reportedly live long lives.

- Meditate to reduce stress. Meditation alters the brain structure through neuro-plasticity, reduces negative thinking, stress and creates calm.
- Change your lifestyle to reduce stress. Change your job, your house, your friends who are toxic. It is up to you, if you have serious cancer you may need to make some drastic changes to beat the odds.
- Drug costs have increased by over 10 percent per year for the last 15 years. In that same period family income has actually declined. Future projections are for drug costs to continue to drive up healthcare costs. This will ensure healthcare is not affordable. Look at alternatives that make sense, talk to your naturopath, be sensible.
- In some parts of the world cancer was not very common. People lived to a ripe old age without developing cancer. We need to research why the increase in cancer rates have occurred and what we can do to reverse these trends. Is it a change in our environment, food additives, increased stress levels? The unifying theory says that it is.
- Instead of having to treat the problem, doesn't it make more sense to prevent it in the first place?

- Donate to medical researchers who are trying to find cancer cures, whether they are patentable or not, not those researchers who are fixated on patents.
- Vote for politicians who want health for all, rather than fiscal health for healthcare corporations and drug companies who lobby them to avoid alternative solutions.

"Factoids"

What follows is a summary of some of the points from the thousands of research papers we analyzed. We have tried to summarize these findings for individuals with a non-science background.

- People who live in certain areas of the world have much lower cancer rates.
- The world cancer research fund reports that "rich" countries have the worst cancer rates, except Japan, which has relatively low rates.
- When groups of people from areas with lower cancer rates move to places with higher rates, such as "developed" countries, their cancer rates increase. This shows that environmental exposure not genes plays the biggest role.
- People who live "cleanly"(no smoking, no alcohol, no treated meat) such as seventh day adventists, have lower cancer rates than other people with similar jobs and exposure to similar environmental toxins.

• Individuals diagnosed with autism have higher rates of cancer.

• On the other hand, individuals diagnosed with psychoses have lower rates of cancer.

• Individuals of the same weight who exercise have lower cancer rates than "couch" potatoes who don't exercise. This indicates that exercise is protective.

• Aerobic exercise helps the gene repair process.

• Vegetarians have lower cancer rates than meat eaters (10-12 percent).

• Micro-environments in areas of the body undergoing cancer metastasis show a lowered (i.e. acidic) pH.

• Warburg in 1920 found that tumors use glycolysis without oxygen to grow, this creates an acid environment.

• Glycolysis (see Warburg) is the breakdown of glucose (sugars).

• Simple sugars are linked to faster cancer growth rates.

• People who avoid high sugar foods are less likely to get cancer.

• Recent studies also show tumors also use fatty acid synthesis for fast growth.

• Fat people are more likely to get cancer than thin people.

• Fat surgery may be a pre cancer preventative technique.

• Cancer cells require energy about 200 times that of normal cells.

• Fat people are more likely to get diabetes.

- The New England Journal of Medicine (2011) reports that people with diabetes have a twenty five percent higher incidence of cancer.
- Diabetics can have acidosis (body levels of acidity that are beyond the normal range). This is due to a drop in insulin levels, more fat burning, glucose levels rising. The ketones from the fat burning raise the acid levels in the blood.
- The level of acidity in a normal human is self regulated, reserves of carbonate in the bones are used to offset high acidity to keep the pH stable.
- There are several mechanisms in the body to ensure pH stability, for example breathing is automatically increased to expel carbon dioxide and decrease acidity.
- The body attempts to control acid levels through more rapid deep breathing to get the carbon dioxide out (acidic breathing).
- Shallow breathing results from stress, increases carbon dioxide in the blood and creates acidosis in the extreme.
- Respiratory acidosis can result from asthma, lung diseases and infections such as pneumonia.
- Asthma patients have taxed immune systems and tend to breathe shallowly, they have higher rates of cancer.
- Acidosis can also result from toxins, alcohol, other drugs, stress and shock.
- Acidosis is indicated as being potentially an indicator of pre-cancer.

- Yogi's use and recommend types of deep breathing to calm the person. This pranayama can reduce carbon dioxide in the blood and induce calm and a sense of well being.
- Yogi's exercise daily, are usually vegetarian and use breath control and as a group are reportedly less likely to get cancer.
- Recent reports show over 60 percent of Americans are overweight or obese.
- The Centre for Disease Control reports that over 20 million Americans have diabetes and that Americans have a one in three chance of becoming diabetic. Five million of them will get cancer.
- Antibodies used for increasing immunity to cancer also decrease asthma severity. Severe asthma often causes acidosis, asthma sufferers are more likely to get cancer.
- Cell death is a normal phenomenon, new cells are created and old ones die, called apoptosis, inside the cell acidity increases in the process of death. Cancer cells seem immune to the acidity.
- Areas of inflammation are more prone to cancer. For example, Crohn's disease patients are more susceptible to certain cancers.
- People with hives and asthma are found to have a higher incidence of leukemia later in life.
- There are 121 million people with depression worldwide,about 10 percent of the population in developed countries.

• Depending on the source from 6 to 15 percent of people in developed countries are addicted to prescription and non-prescription drugs and alcohol.

• Millions of people have low levels of vitamin D and are thought to be immune compromised.

• Most people do not eat a well balanced diet with vegetables (such as broccoli) proven to reduce susceptibility to cancer.

• Cancer cells need a blood supply to live.They use more energy than normal cells. Cutting off their blood supply is effective.

• Studies have shown a decrease in normal blood hemoglobin levels lead up to a cancer diagnosis.

• Cancer cells have fewer defenses than normal cells and die more easily, if you can get to them. That is why many therapies work without maiming the patient.

• Intravenous vitamin C at high levels in a petri dish and presumably in the blood can help reduce the formation of new blood supplies to cancer cells and can kill cancer cells by apoptosis (CMAJ study).

• Chemicals isolated from cruciferous vegetables have been found to cause apoptosis (cell death) in cancer cells by changing gene expression, without affecting normal cells.

• Shift workers are more likely to get both diabetes and cancer. This is thought to be as a result of the stress of changing circadian rhythms. The pineal gland produces melatonin to regulate biological rhythms.

• Melatonin levels are higher when you are young. Cancer is more likely when you are old.

• Melatonin therapy reduces death rates in those with cancer.

• Melatonin has a protective influence on mitochondria and gene repair at a cellular level.

• Mitochondria generate energy and help regulate cell death (remember, cancer cells use more energy).

• Cancer patients who have recovered, have no tumors and normal blood work often report chronic fatigue.

• Gene defects in mitochondria are thought to contribute to many diseases of the elderly possibly including cancer.

• Stress causes adrenaline which has now been found to accelerate tumor growth in cancer patients.

• Recent cell phone studies find no link between cell phone use and cancer for the average user, but did find a small effect for heavy users of cell phones, indicating that stress related use may be additive.

• Cancer stem cells have been found in several types of cancer and are now thought to be present in all cancers.

• Radiation and chemotherapy kill normal cancer cells but apparently not the cancer stem cells so targeting the stem cells is becoming a major research initiative.

• Toxins (such as the chemicals in cigarette smoke) cause genetic mutations.

• The body has self correcting mechanisms to repair the genes. If these mechanisms fail cancer cells proliferate.

- Cell mutations occur at the rate of between 1,000 and 1,000,000 per day. Understanding the repair mechanism is a key research area in cancer research.
- Telomeres are the tips of chromosomes and when shortened and affected by an enzyme can lead to cancer. Stress has been hypothesized as the cause of the enzyme-shortening issue which affects the telomeres and prompts cancer. This may be a genetic-stress link in the cancer model.
- Medical baseline research is based on “normal” medical student volunteers who are healthy and active. These people are actually not normal, they are the extremely healthy and well educated. We need more research on the real normal.
- The real profile of a “normal” person in developed countries is, a person with one or more of the following attributes; overweight, pre diabetic and inactive, depressed, possibly with allergies, asthma and infections complaining of stress and addictions.
- The war on cancer is slowly working. There are a few designer drugs that cause complete remission. The majority of cancers do not have such solutions yet. In the interim we need to get everyone working together for the benefit of the patients. This needs serious consideration of the unifying theory and a commitment for all health professionals to work as a team to help patients beat the odds.

To conclude: *Cancer is a result of psychological, physiological, metabolic and spiritual stress.*

Reducing all stress is necessary to create an environment where cancer will not proliferate. The addition of supplements, improved diet and exercise will help to induce cancer cell death.

Continuing with stress reduction and a solid cancer fighting strategy will help to reduce reoccurrence of the cancer.

Appendix One - Unifying Theory

APPENDIX TWO-Resources

Here are some internet resources to get you started. Each website is a portal to a huge amount of other information. Note, the author does not receive any commission for including any of these links. Please note this is only a partial list of sites that offer health information. All of these sites offer their information free of charge which is why these sources of excellent health information have been recommended.

General Cancer information

American Cancer Society	**www.cancer.org**
Australian Cancer Council	**www.cancer.org.au**
Canadian Cancer society	**www.cancer.ca/**
Cancer Index	**www.cancerindex.org/**
Cancer Care Ontario	**www.cancercare.on.ca/**
Medical Dictionary-NIH-Medline	**www.nlm.nih.govmedlineplus/ mplusdictionary.html**
Pubmed (NIH)	**www.ncbi.nlm.nih.gov/pubmed/**
National Coalition for Cancer Survivorship	**www.canceradvocacy.org/**
Mayo Clinic	**www.mayoclinic.com/health-information/**
New Zealand Cancer Society	**www.cancernz.org.nz/**

UK Cancer Centres **www.cancerindex.org/clink44r.htm**

US National Library of Medicine PubMed www.ncbi.nlm.nih.gov/sites/entrez?db=pubmed

UK Cancer Index **www.cancerindex.org/clinks1.htm**

UK National Institute for Health and Clinical Excellence. **www.nice.org.uk**

Note the medical dictionary is really key to understanding many of the terms used and our suggestion is that you keep it open in the background as you do your research.

Pubmed is the main internet source for evidence based articles on any health issue, keep in mind that even these sources are sometimes suspect, see chapter one for more information.

Health Alerts

Google alerts can be found at **www.google.com/alerts**

Food/Diet Resources

Pubmed is the best place to search for articles on specific foods and to check out whether something is being oversold by those with financial links to products.

One of the largest cancer studies to date has been the EPIC study in Europe. This study has confirmed many of the findings mentioned in the Unifying theory. To read more go to: **www.epic.iarc.fr**

Perhaps the best book we have read on cancer fighting foods is "Foods That Fight Cancer" by Gingras and Beliveau, researchers in Montreal. Go to **www.richardbeliveau.org** .

Other books that focus on fighting cancer and healthy eating:

Anti cancer: A New Way of Life, David Servan-Schreiber, MD PhD, Harper Collins, 2007.

Prescription for Nutritional Healing- Fourth Edition, Phyllis A. Balch, Penguin Group 2006.

The Science of Good Food, David Joachim and Andrew Schloss, Robert Rose Publishing, 2008.

The Food Connection, Sam Graci, Macmillian Publishing 2001.

The End of Food: How the Food Industry is Destroying our Food Supply & What We Can Do About It, Thomas F. Pawlick, Greystone Books, 2006.

Good Cook Books for Cancer Fighting Diets

Here is a list of cook books that Elizabeth found helpful when she was trying to make a change from traditional North American meat based cooking to more cancer flighting cooking. The recipes in these cook books helped us to make the transition to a larger proportion of vegetarian meals. These cookbooks were inspiring and the dishes in them were not only healthy but they were gastronomically awesome.

Beliveau R., and Gingras D.,, "Cooking with Foods That Fight Cancer", McClelland and Stewart Ltd.

Katzen Mollie, " The New Moosewood Cookbook", Ten Speed Press

Lawrence N., "The Dao of Harmony Dawn Cooking",www.harmonydawn.com.

Lawrence N. and James A., Eco Harmony Dawn Cooking, Balancing Your internal and External Environments, www.harmonydawn.com.

Salomon and Jolar, "Hollyhock Cooks", www.newsociety.com.

Exercise

Get off that couch!!! Ok I'll stop shouting!

Pubmed is the best place for research, just enter the form of exercise and the word cancer. For example the search entitled "Yoga Cancer" revealed 103 articles. Try making the searches very general like this to start, then becoming more specific. The search for Yoga Pranayama Cancer only had 2 articles.

Check with a medical expert before doing exercise during or after treatment.

Here is the link for Gary Bello's Yoga DVD which we use and have used since my treatments, it worked for me;

www.gopalgarybello.com/products/dvd-yoga.html

Psychology/Spirituality

This part is up to you depending on your religious beliefs, and whether you can afford to hire a psychologist or not. Even if you have no money you may find clinics that will offer pro bono counseling or volunteer groups like Wellspring (www.wellspring.ca). Churches and community groups are always willing to help or to suggest someone who can.

Don't make the mistake of believing you can do it yourself. Denial is not just a river in Egypt. Be brave, ask for help. Many of these websites will put you in contact with helplines, forums, organizations and individuals if they cannot directly help you themselves, all are free:

Cancerbackup -UK	www.cancerbackup.org.uk
Cancer Research UK	www.cancerhelp.org.uk
The Haven breast cancer centres	www.thehaven.org.uk
MacMillan Cancer Support-UK	www.macmillan.org.uk
Maggie's centres UK	www.maggiescentres.org

Marie Curie Cancer care UK	www.mariecurie.org.uk
National Institutes of Mental Health -US	www.nimh.nih.gov
Wellspring (Canada)	www.welspring.ca
Cancer forums	www.cancerforums.net
Cancer Mentors	www.4thangel.org
Cancer Support Community	www.cancersupportcommunity.org
Livestrong (formerly Lance Armstrong)	www.livestrong.org
Imerman Angels-Mentors	www.imermanangels.org
Support and Online Counseling	www.cancercare.org
Australian Countrywide Online Support	www.lifeline.org.au
Australian Cancer Council Helpline	www.cancervic.org.au

APPENDIX THREE-Allan Hirsh Emails

This appendix will give you a sampling of one persons ups and downs from just after diagnosis to the end of treatment. It is included because Allan is both funny and honest about his emotions. People who have read this said it was healing for them.

This story is a sampling of the almost daily interchange between Allan Hirsh, cartoonist and Michael from October 2010 to November 2011. Michael's words have been edited out for the most part to keep it brief, what he said is obvious based on Allan's questions or responses.

We are happy to report that Allan is well and happy!

- I have been reading Anti-cancer; a new way of life by Dr. Servan-Schrieiber, MD, PhD.

  Reading about how cancer develops and the natural defenses of the body has been fascinating. I have been really enjoying realizing how incredible the body is at self-regulation. When I read his chapters on the importance of positive attitude and the role of food in maintaining health and balance, I feel very positive and empowered.

  I have a naturopath in North Bay who I trust and have started working with her. Last year she helped me lower my blood pressure. I look forward to hearing about your journey.

- I have just read most of Life Over Cancer; The Block Center Program for Integrative Cancer Treatment.

  The more I understand, the more in control of the process I feel, even though I am actually only a raft on a river clinging to faith and will.I am ready for the challenge.....and some more green tea.Light, love, laughter and healing.

- From what I have read, helplessness and loneliness appears to make recovery harder. Empowerment and a positive attitude seem to prolong life. There are many stories of individuals with terminal cancer who began to meditate daily and achieved a complete recovery. I have been meditating twice daily. Some meditations are deeper than others; others not so deep. The other night, mind you, I had a dream in which I was able to fill my head and body with bright, white light. I then walked outside and felt totally in the present moment, celebrating life in myself and all that was around me.

  I know that I am more than my body. Most of the time I have been in a pretty good space, focusing on what I want to achieve and what I can do to heal, instead of my fears of what could happen if events don't go well. I have been reading and absorbing information about the body at an intensity I have not experienced since I worked on my master's degree. Joan has been cooking up a therapeutic storm using fresh organic vegetables, turmeric, ginger, garlic, pepper and olive oil. Add a lot of green tea and a touch of dark chocolate and voila; a healthy, healing feast that at the very least makes me feel content and loved.

- Radiation will probably not kill all the cancer cells. It will be up to me to help my body reclaim its ability to maintain wellness and a positive outcome. As I write these words, I feel up to the challenge. I am still waiting, however, for the Sudbury Cancer Treatment Centre to call me with a schedule. I am trying not to anticipate, but I can't really schedule much unless I know where I stand. I have only been seeing a few clients a week and have not been accepting new clients. I was at film club last night, watching "Get Low" (which was an excellent film with Robert Duvall). Within the first forty minutes I had to pee three times. I know everyone was watching the movie and not me, but somehow I felt oddly exposed and vulnerable.
- Some people know about my cancer and have been really caring and supportive. I am reluctant to tell every acquaintance I meet, however, because it doesn't seem appropriate to do that. Yet I feel like I am putting a false wall when they ask me how I am and I say today is a good day

  One study that I read compared breast cancer survival rates with women who had ten friends vs women who did not. The group with friends had a much better survival rate.So thank you for being part of this story.
- I will welcome the radiation into my body with love as it attacks those pesky cancer cells.

I have been given African drumming music to listen to on my MP3 player during the actual radiation. Apparently, sound vibrations can be helpful during treatment. I will give that a try. I would even wear a blue dress if I thought it might help. Not any blue dress, however. The colour would have to match my eyes.

Yes, I am going to Sudbury which is about a one and half hour drive on a good day. Fortunately, I have a four wheel drive car with good snow tires.

I am seeing my Naturopath on Monday and will get some probiotics then (is that the same as biotics?)

She will also inject me with mistletoe which will make me good to hang around at Christmas time. Modified fruit pectin, pumpkin seed, ground flax, ginger, garlic, and green tea will help out as well.I will stop taking extra vit C.. and E during radiation because the oncologist asked me to. When I looked into the research the results are conflicting so I will hold off during the course of treatment and then pile it on afterwards. I am reading Quantum Healing which reinforces my belief in the power of mind and spirit to heal.

- I didn't put it in my PPP,(Allan refers to his support group as PPP) but on Friday I saw my Reiki therapist who is quite intuitive and wonderfully,lovingly, cosmically flaky.

  She had a whole list of instructions which were quite helpful. She suggested I put my hands over my heart chakra when I feel fear and sing when I need to.

She pointed out that I am undergoing a transformation and to not worry about money because all will work out.
She said I need to rest and to avoid people who will drain me.
She said to welcome the radiation lovingly and it will help me.
So will peppermint tea.

- I feel hopeful about the outcome. I am just a little anticipatory about the day to day. Yesterday, I spent time with my two year old grandson and we had a blast.I want to see this fellow as a teenager.

- I drove to Sudbury through a blizzard this morning. I briefly thought that running into a transport truck would not advance my healing so I slowed down. The snow eventually turned to rain. Not long after that a work crew was stopping traffic on the highway. The woman with the stop sign smiled and waved at everyone. Most travelers seemed to wave back at her sunshine.

- I have been getting gas at an Esso station half way between North Bay and Sudbury. The owner is a very friendly East Indian man who always greats me with a smile even if I am only there sometimes to use the washroom. I also discovered a store on the highway called Neat Stuff which actually had some neat stuff. Everything flowed wonderfully today (after the snow passed) and I enjoyed talking to everyone I met. Only 39 days of traveling left, but who is counting.

- Vancouver is 4,000 km from North Bay. Each round trip to Sudbury and back is 262 km.This means that 41 days of traveling for treatment is equivalent to driving from North Bay to Vancouver and back again and then heading out to the east Coast.

- The highway to Sudbury is in fairly good condition. The scenery is pretty in parts and interesting in others. Sudbury used to look like a moonscape. Acid rain from Sudbury's tall mining smokestacks had killed most of the vegetation. In recent years, however, with new filters on the smokestacks, vegetation has begun to cling to the rocks. The landscape is still pretty dramatic and harsh in parts. Sudbury is a rich mining area because the city lies in a basin that was created when a large meteor fell to the earth before mankind was even created.
- I actually have been enjoying my drives back and forth, listening to the radio or to music or talking with my occasional co-pilot. Today, George, an old dear friend helped me drive. Yesterday, Joan, took the wheel part of the way.
- Despite the beauty of the drive, or the grace of having a loving friend next to me, the urge to pee can take precedence. Radiation irritates tissue, which make me want to pee even more than usual. I met a prostate cancer survivor in the swimming pool today. He had a PSA of 2500 and has been alive 14 years after receiving radiation. He said that he has peed under most of the trees in northern Ontario. He also said that from his experience, attitude predicts survival.

- The trouble with needing to pee so often (if you can excuse me for always coming back to this point) is that it makes sleeping through the night difficult. This leads, of course to fatigue,
- I was very tired today until I started my radiation. I lay there listening to some music a yoga teacher gave me, watching my breath rise and fall. After a while I began to see light flowing through my body with every breath. I felt invigorated after the session. I really, really had to pee, but I felt invigorated and hopeful.
- I was reading the other day that there are documented cases of multiple personality (now known as dissociative disorder) where one personality (alter) can have a cold, while a different alter of the same person remains healthy. One alter can have allergies, but not the others. In one case I read about, one alter tested positive for colour blindness, while the others didn't. To me this speaks to the power of the mind over the body. Change the personality and the body changes with it.
- Did you know that cancer patients who have support from friends and family tend to live longer? Now is a good time to thank all of you for being there and giving me the opportunity to share my journey with you. I am finding this process very helpful to me and it is becoming an important part of my healing.
- I listen to pain all day long as part of my work. People ask me how I am able do such a thing day in and day out. I am a karma yogi. This means that I can get lost by serving others. It can

bring me joy to do so. I can also see possible positive outcomes that others often can't. To set aside most of my practice and ask others for help is new to me.

- To share my vulnerabilities is somewhat frightening, yet I have been reassured by your steadfastness and responses in this process.
- In October of 2009, my mother had a stroke one day before her 90th birthday party. She passed away six months later. Since then I have spoken to my 92 year old father almost every morning. He was there for my mother for 66 years for better or for worse. He supported her in the last months of her life with a strength and consistency that moved me. He has had cancer three times and continues to carry on with the business of life.On Friday morning he reported experiencing so much pain that he could hardly move.
- He went to the hospital in Montreal and my brother Harvey stood by his side through the diagnostic process. Was he dying? If he was, could I go visit him? Could I postpone my radiation to go to the funeral? I definitely felt helpless and heavy. On one hand I know I need to generate positive energy to heal, but on the other hand I need to feel authentic emotions as part of the healing process as well.
- I drove to Sudbury today with a heavy heart. The weather was really, really foggy. There was hardly any visibility at all. I kept my eyes on the taillights a head of me and on the highway lines that defined the road. The road became my meditation and took

my mind away from all my weariness. Not long after I returned home, I heard from my father for the first time in three days. I was very relieved to speak to him. It turns out his cancer has spread into the tenth vertebrae in his spine. His oncologist has set up some radiation for him and sent him home with some pain killers. He is one month away from moving into an assisted living home. I am pretty sure now that he will be able to follow through on his plans. He has had radiation before and breezes through it.

- When I built my house so many years ago, I was totally preoccupied with the project. Building is about measuring, cutting, carrying and nailing over and over again.Gradually, a wall is completed...then another and another. Working on the second floor only means that now everything has to be carried up a ladder. At first my mind would wonder and shout to me about fatigue or black flies or back aches, but eventually I was able to work with a more peaceful mind, focused in the moment on the task at hand.
- I realize that I am using the same approach with my encounter with cancer. Each day, each meal, each drive to Sudbury, I am taking another step to wellness and recovery.It is hard to generate at lot of cosmic healing energy when you are exhausted, but I did manage to meditate during the radiation session. Somehow, I was able to visualize a peaceful purple light. I am not sure what this means, but it did feel good.

- I returned home to discover that the ministry of health has denied my travel grant allowance because they did not receive a referral from my urologist. I, of course, had sent them a referral from my urologist and will now have to do the paper work all over again.The paperwork is redundant, mind you, because you can't get treatment at the Cancer Centre without a referral. The rush of anger that I felt towards the indifferent bureaucrat who sent me the refusal did perk my energy up for a moment or two.
- The radiation machine that I use is number four. I studied math for five years at the same time I studied psychology. Some numbers speak positively to me for some reason. I like the number four. On December 13th, it will be retired and eventually replaced by a newer model. This process will take six months. Much of the cement wall surrounding number four will have to be rebuilt and anything that may have absorbed stray radiation will be removed. I will be switched to an odd numbered machine. I hope to adjust to this change, or will this be the event which finally propels me into a rocking fetus position.I will let you know if this occurs, as well as any concurrent therapeutic value in such an exercise.

  Possible advantages of retreating into a fetus position.

  - It can be oddly comforting and restful
  - Young children will identify and even begin to climb over you
  - Household heating costs can come down slightly

- It is reminiscent of your first high school or freshman year university hangover
- It can be distracting if you add rocking behaviour

Disadvantages of the fetus position.

- It can pick up dust and carpet lint
- It is difficult to drive a car
- It is not very warrior like
- It does not instill confidence in your abilities as a therapist
- It makes it even harder to get up and pee

- I did some pranayama today which felt good. My friend who is a Shiatso therapist is coming to visit for a couple of days....just in time I must say.
- The other day a man came up to me at the YMCA Peace Week celebrations and asked if I wanted to hear a joke. I always say yes to such a question. He described a minister who told his flock that everyone in his congregation was destined to die and be judged. This elicited an outburst of laughter from a man in the front row. The minister asked him why he was laughing. The man replied that he was from another congregation and was only visiting. Somewhat dark, but I did like this joke.
- Last night was my roughest night yet. My rear end was burning and the urge to pee was relentless. I have taught pain management strategies so I started working through a few.
- Witness the pain without judging the sensations as pain. Well, I could call the pain tapioca pudding, but it still wasn't pleasant.

I did some Yoga deep breathing exercises which helped for a while, but the night is longer than a while. I actually did try rocking in a fetal position, but I found it overrated. My fear was that the pain would continue and get worse over the coming weeks. At three in the morning, I slipped out of bed and began to watch the Steven Spielberg HBO miniseries about World War Two in the Pacific.

This is a story of young men who fought in horrible conditions against all odds. I had previously watched the first miniseries called Band of Brothers which moved me deeply. The stories depicted in the Band of Brothers and the The Pacific are based on real characters and events. How did these young men find the strength and courage to continue on? After watching a few minutes of the first segment, my situation did not seem as bad as it did. I am in a battle of a different sort, but one I plan to win.

At about four in the morning I had a terrible case of diarrhea. After that, thankfully, the pain subsided and I was able to actually fall asleep for a while. The morning is looking brighter and more hopeful. Thank you for hanging in there with me.

- In my head, I am aware of a lifetime of subliminal messages. Be Strong. Don't show weakness, Don't complain. Be a man.
- I am sure that many people have had to put up with much more severe symptoms for a longer period of time. Am I weak because it is bothering me so much?

I usually enjoy my body. I love exercising and how it feels to stretch, relax and move my body. I can tolerate back pain, muscles aches, even everything I went through to get diagnosed. I don't like fatigue and I don't like stomach cramps. I think part of the problem is that I am projecting that these symptoms will get worse and not better.

I have also based part of my self-esteem on what I can accomplish in a day. Now my main challenge is whether or not I can make it to the bathroom in time.

- Fortunately, two of my dear long term friends have come up north for a brief visit. Marc is a G.P. Psychotherapist who has been a mentor and a subversive humourist who actually gets most of my attempts at wit. JoAnne is an incredibly warm person who is both a music teacher and an experienced Shiatso practitioner. Last night she gave me a one hour treatment in which I saw white light and felt my body relax. I slept well for most of the night and glimpsed normality again. This suggests to me that I need to keep my spiritual energy up by doing yoga, meditating and deep breathing.

  During the radiation, I was able to visualize a wonderful blue light which energized me and helped me feel hopeful.

- Michael, I have always been a good karma yogi but not so good at sitting and meditating. I am working on it, but two hours is way beyond me at this point.

  I can barely watch two hours of TV.

In order to pee sometimes I visualize a flowing river like the last chapter in Sidhartha. Poignant, but not really meditation.

- There are two parts of the trip where traffic comes to a complete halt for road construction. I mentioned earlier, that there was a woman who flags the traffic down and then mouths have a nice day as she waves you on your journey with a smile. She doesn't need to be so friendly, but her positive energy is infectious. Many of the cancer patients I have met who travel the highway have commented on her. Everyone waves back at her. Today, she was flagging right near the Warren Esso station where I make a regular half way stop. I bought a five dollar bag of chocolate candies and walked out onto the highway and gave it to her. I said this is from all of the travelers at the Sudbury Cancer Center. We really appreciate your positive attitude. She took the candies and beamed a little brighter. Those few moments, made my day.
- Despite being up much of the night with a persistent urge to pee, my day wasn't too bad at all. I saw my oncologist today. When she asked how I was, I told her that if I had a dollar for every time I peed, I would be a wealthy man. She said that she didn't have any money for me, but she did give me a prescription for Flowmax. What a name for a drug. I could picture myself writing my full name in snow. If there are any side effects, the information brochure suggests that I should contact my doctor, pharmacist, biographer and plumber. The drug, apparently will have little effect for a week or so. In the

meantime, I told the doctor that I have been visualizing a river or waterfall to help myself relax during urination. The doctor suggested that putting one hand in warm water would help. I returned home to discover that the bathroom sink is six feet away from the toilet bowel. I am not sure how to get around this, yet.

- The Block Integrative Cancer treatment program at Northwestern University (Life Over Cancer) says that green tea actually supports the work of the radiation.

Yesterday was a good day. The oncologist said that the diarrhea would end soon after the first 25 more intense radiation treatments ended. The idea of the side effects ending at some point was quite encouraging. Feeling good, I went to the Y for a relaxing swim and a stretch in the hot therapeutic pool. I forgot that chlorine and heat are not recommended during radiation treatment. I woke up at three in the morning with a strong burning sensation that just would not go away. As of 10:00 this morning, after seeing my naturopath, I had stocked up with a long list of medicinal tools and ointments. They did not help last night, mind you. At 4:00am, I lay in bed, repeating my meditation mantra over and over, focusing above my chin to the best of my ability. Eventually, I did fall asleep and woke up pain free two hours later.

I did have another treatment in Sudbury today. My friend Terry drove there and back because I really was too tired to fully concentrate on the road. Today was my thirteenth treatment.

The first treatment segment is more than half way over. Today was my treatment Bar Mitzfa. Elliah Moisha (my Hebrew name).

- Today, the roller coaster ride was actually pleasant. I slept fairly well and was even able to go for a workout at the Y this morning. No, I did not go swimming.

  My oldest North Bay friend, George, drove me to Sudbury today. We listened to an old Cat Stevens CD. The music took us back to the sixties and a time of expansion, fluidity, growth and spiritual imagination. This afternoon, we were on a road trip again, visiting our youth and transcending the limits of our situation. Some of what we learned in our younger, freer days has helped us become the creative professionals that we are, able to see past many of the boxes and limiting labels that greet us each day. Today was not a day of illness, but a day of celebration.

- Every second day or so there is a "new normal". This can consist of a new sensation or discomfort or an old familiar pain. It all comes down to accepting what is unfolding and finding someway to deal with it.

  I had previously mentioned that I was refused a daily travel grant allowance that I am entitled to. I have since resubmitted the appropriate doctor signed forms. I also included a letter to the person who refused my initial application at the Ministry of Health and Long term Care. I enjoyed writing the letter and have included a copy of part of it below.

"I do not expect you to care that I have prostate cancer or that I have to drive the equivalent of a return cross-Canada trip. I also do not expect you to empathize with my fatigue or pain or the fact that I can not work right now. I do expect you to do your job in such a way that my life is made easier because of you, not harder.So many patients that I have spoken to do not question your department's denial of funding because they are too tired, frustrated, or too confused to do so.

I look forward to seeing my checks in the future. It is far cheaper for the Ministry to pay for travel than to actually build treatment facilities that are more accessible."

- Yesterday, I was able to relax and take some time to continue reading Deepak Chopra's Quantum Healing. He talked about the healing qualities of bliss, which I am all in favour of. Go bliss, go! He also talked about remembering that most of the body, aside from the cancer, is healthy and functioning well. It really is a hopeful, empowering book.

  It was really disappointing, however, to discover that a burning irritation and the need to pee every fifteen minutes has come to visit me again. Sleep was hard and sparse. Fortunately, Joan was able to drive me to Sudbury today, while I rested. The drive home was painful for me because of the aforementioned condition. Corn silk tea and cranberry juice did not seem to help(yet). Taking an aspirin somehow allows me to sit and write. At the end of this week, I will be halfway through my total radiation program. Is my schedule half full or half empty? Either way, forward we go.

- Good answer, Michael! In Deepak's book, he talks about the brain being the central processor of all sensory information. Reality rests in our perception.
- In the middle of my evening pilgrimages, my son Jacob called to see how I was doing. Just talking to him seemed to calm me down. The calmer I became, the less urgency I had to pee. Jacob is going for a job interview at Harvard tomorrow. He calmed me down and helped change my focus. I think I helped him center as well. I slept very well last night.

  In the morning I picked up the medication that was prescribed and dropped off my sample at the hospital lab. I ran into an old client with an overnight bag. He seemed quite nervous and out of sorts. He was there for surgery on his prostate. He was afraid he would panic because he had to stay in one place for quite a while. I told him he would only panic if he wanted to maintain a semblance of control. All he had to do was surrender his dignity and privacy and let his doctor do his work. I also told him that it would be alright. He laughed and was visibly relieved after our encounter. It did not feel like an accident that I ran into him.
- I arrived in Sudbury an hour early today was surprised that they called me for radiation right after I arrived. I quickly drank down my pre-radiation cup of peppermint tea only to discover that there were three people ahead of me. To make a

long, painful story short, I almost peed on the radiation table. I guess it happens a lot.

It is so strange that at this point of my healing, everything comes down to the timing, nature, and ability to pee. All this could be embarrassing and humiliating if I didn't know that so many others are in the same situation as I. Having been able to broach this subject with all of you, has helped mc become more accepting of this predicament. Or, as my dear writer friend, Phil has said: just go with the flow and don't push the river.

In the last few pages of Sidhartha by Herman Hesse, a young Buddha discovers that the river of life is everywhere and always continues to flow. Yes, I could end now with that poignant reference, but I just wanted to add that the medication I just started taking turns my urine bright (and I mean bright)...orange.

- Thanks for the encouragement, Michael. Tell me, did your PSA come down after treatment? Were you able to pee better after treatment? Did you grow a green tail?I finished reading Deepak Chopra's book "Quantum Healing". He gives example after example of how the will to live can restart the natural healing abilities of the body. Within my DNA is a complete blueprint for my very existence. It is very detailed and incredibly complex. In my meditation and prayers I am trying to nudge my DNA into full healing mode. Faith and will seem to be quite powerful, but Dr. Chopra talks about the power of bliss which he defines as a joyous, altered form of consciousness that transcends our day to day limited view of reality. I have experienced this in the past and have been glimpsing this in the guise of love more and more often. Joan has been looking really good these days. That may be a result of this love consciousness I am working on.

- Thank you once again, Michael. I think when we surrender to healing we are accessing what Deepak calls bliss. May the entire world experience bliss.
- I was pretty tired by the time I was called for my treatment. The sessions begin with an ultrasound of my bladder and prostate to make sure that my bladder is full enough and to locate my prostate which tends to move around between treatments. As I lie there, two radiation technicians look through my pubic hair for a previously tattooed dot. When found, the dot becomes the center of a large cross that the radiation machine will focus on. It is difficult to make appropriate small talk when two attractive women are looking through your pubic hair with intense focused attention. When they leave the room, I am to lie totally still until directed otherwise. The table I am on, rises about four feet into the air. I have already chosen music which plays in the background. I close my eyes and either rest or meditate on my body becoming healthier and stronger. After the session, it is imperative that I find an empty washroom quickly.
- The radiated northern ice trucker prepares for yet another adventure. Boots, blankets, bananas, water bottle, warm layers

of clothing, candles, matches, scarves and a snow shovel. Check. Inner resolve, determination, focus, positive intent and, for today, a lovely co-pilot named Joan who has proven herself in winter storms time and time again. Check. A full tank of gas in preparation for the journey. But, alas, control once again proves to be illusive as it slips away, for yet another day. The local radio station is quite insistent; the highway from North Bay to Sturgeon Falls and beyond is closed due to white out and icy conditions. A major accident involving several big vehicles is blocking the highway. The longer, detour route is also closed because of five semi trailers that ran into each other. There is nothing to do, but surrender. The missed day of radiation will be added at the end.

- While I was waiting for treatment, I ran into three of the men who I had previously met. The oldest of the three said "Oh, oh. Here comes trouble" as he looked up at me. I told him to be careful because I brought my muscle with me and then nodded to Terry. The second fellow struck me as a retired miner who was grumpy a lot. It turns out he was a retired minister which totally surprised me somehow. The third man talked symptoms and how many treatments we both had left. I somehow feel connected to these guys who are sharing a similar journey with me. I gave each of them a homemade cartoon Christmas card which brought smiles to their faces. I liked that.
- When I studied the psychology of animal behaviour in University, I came across a research theory called Hull's Goal

Gradient Hypothesis. It has been observed that a rat in a maze will begin to speed up the closer it gets to the final goal. I feel a little like that rat. I want to move things along, but I still have to trundle on one day at a time, one hour at a time, one moment at a time. I felt low energy this morning, but had to visit my office to pick up some mail and pay some bills. I ran into eight people I know. I received some hugs, smiles, a Christmas present and some really caring wishes for health. That really helped.

- George, a colleague and friend, drove me to Sudbury. We had a good time discussing everything under the sun from philosophy to psychology. On the way back, I slipped into the Tim Horton's at Sturgeon Falls to pee (of course) and to order a plain, toasted, 12 grain bagel. Now please allow me to digress for a moment. About the same time that I was studying about Hull and his research, I was living with four other students above Pine's Pizza shop in Montreal. Our apartment was around the corner from a Hari Krishna temple and was ten minutes away from McGill University. It was a perfect place to live in the late sixties. I do admit to inhaling and exhaling herbs that were quite common at that time. Sometimes, late at night, we would all have the urge to eat large quantities of pizza. We were not always lucid enough to march downstairs and order the pizza with a straight face. One day, we sent Jack downstairs to order the pizza. He was trying really hard to stay focused and appear normal. Without Jack knowing, we all snuck downstairs and waited for Jack to enter the restaurant. Just as he was about to open his mouth to order, we all surprised him by jumping in front of the restaurant's window with absurd expressions on our faces. The clerk had his back to us and had no idea why Jack collapsed in a total fit of laughter. Jack was not able to recover for at least an hour and we didn't get to have pizza that night. Which brings me back to my bagel at Tim Hortons. Just as I was about to place my order, I notice George standing absolutely still, in the corner window, staring at me with a totally serious look on his face. I immediately flashed back to the Pine's Pizza event and began to laugh. The clerk, to her credit, laughed along with me, even though she had no idea what I was laughing at. George moved from window to window while I attempted to avoid a total eruption of hilarity.

There are only 12 more treatments left. I am tired, but I am not sure if that is because of the radiation, the routine or a side effect of the medication I am on (or all three). Everyone who sees me tells me how good I look. I am not sure if I actually look good or that people are expecting me to look like I am on death's door.

I like the Holiday Season because everyone is a little friendlier than usual. I wish all of you health, light and love; perhaps even some peace and joy. I thank you all for sharing this journey with me and giving of yourselves with your presence and caring.

Om shanti. Shalom Aleichem. Om mani padme hum. Merry Christmas

- I read that if your sports team wins your testosterone will increase; if your team loses your hormones will decrease. So please, choose sports teams that lose. Also, sell your BMW if you have one.

  “A wise man should consider that his health is the greatest of human blessings and learn how, by his own thought, to derive benefit from his illnesses. “Hippocrates

  This last year has brought challenges and growth. I want to thank all of you for being part of this unfolding. Your encouragement, shared perspectives and energy have helped me immensely. I wish you all a Happy New Year with health, peace, joy, light and love. (Only seven more treatments left).

  Michael, a full fledged Prostate Partner, responded to what I wrote yesterday with the following:

  “Scientifically we change every year, new cells replace the old. Deep inside we are the same, what changes is the darkness that the cancer cells represent is gone, our body is at first confused by the loss, then as new non cancer cells develop our body recognizes the youthfulness of it all and everything seems brighter, more alive.”

  I like that.

- I am quite aware that there are many people who have had to struggle harder than I have. In the cancer clinic you meet people in all sorts of predicaments. After all I have been through, I realized I have not seen one damn clown! You would think that somewhere, somehow, someone would have thought to bring a clown on board as part of the treatment team. I guess clowns are only brought in to cheer up kids and not adults who are kids at heart.

- My friend Mike told me of a fellow who was calm in the face of bad news. He was told he only had a few months to live so he systematically began to sell off all of his snow machines and four wheelers. After selling off $60,000 of his toys, he found out that he was in remission. Surprise.
- As I was lying on the radiation table for the LAST time, and as the two young radiation technicians were looking through what is left of my pubic hair for the tattooed target mark, I said: " God forbid, but if I ever have to go through this again, I am going to have a tattoo of a happy face. " The two women cracked up which was a good thing.On my drive home, I pulled into the Esso station at Warren. I have stopped at this station twice a day for 41 days. I have probably bought over a $1,000 worth of gas. Kap, the Hindu gentleman who owns the station, has always greeted me with a warm smile and well wishes. He has been counting down the days with me. I gave him a copy of my book (Relax for the Fun of It) and thanked him for his positive energy. To my surprise, he gave me a gift bag containing a very large chocolate bar and a birthday card. We shook hands and wished me well; such a nice man. He made

me feel so comfortable even when I was running into his place, desperate to pee.

- So here I am at the end of the radiation and the incessant traveling. I am grateful I have made it this far in tact. The next step in my journey of healing must continue, however. My follow up appointment is in North Bay on April 20. The radiation had cleansed my body hopefully of all the cancer cells. I must now engage the intelligence of my body to continue to cleanse me of cancer cells. Through diet, supplements, meditation, attitude, laughter, prayer, exercise, purpose, faith, will and love I will move forward to health and wellness.I had read that cancer patients who felt empowered, hopeful and supported tended to do well. I formed the Positive Prostate Partnership to keep me on track and to help me remember who I am and what I am capable of. I feel like I have come through this experience connected to my deeper self as well as connected to all of you. I feel deep love, appreciation and gratitude. Thank you all.
- It has been three weeks since my last radiation treatment. So far, I have received thirty Northern Health Travel Grant checks for $61.50; each one in a separate envelope. It seems a little inefficient to me, but I am happy to receive the checks. I am definitely battling fatigue. My energy level is still below par. I have been seeing clients, but only two to four a day. I will no longer work nights or work on Fridays.

I seem to have lost some of my protective wall that comes in handy when dealing with hostile clients. I saw a couple who were arguing over their six year old daughter and her bed wetting problem. The step-father was angry at the young girl and wanted to punish her each and every time she wet the bed. I found myself identifying with the young girl and the mounting pressure on her to pee appropriately. Within twenty minutes of the start of the session, I felt a strong urge to pee. I excused myself and experienced a burning sensation reminiscent of two months ago. Twenty minutes later the same thing happened. I handled the session well and I think I helped the couple get to a kinder and better strategy for dealing with the girl, but I felt that I had worked really hard. When I got home, I took one of those pills that turn my pee bright orange and the irritation subsided. I am grateful that the irritation has not returned since.

- I was talking to a fellow at the YMCA who survived prostate cancer. His PSA remained the same for a while but then became lower as soon as he changed his diet. This made me feel hopeful and reinforced the diet aspect of my anti-cancer approach. I remain yours, steadfastly in recovery, with faith and love.
- It has been quite a while since I have written. I find that I do miss writing. It is a way to center myself and put my feelings and thoughts in order (or, at the very least, behind me). It has been about a week short of three months since my last radiation

treatment.My shamanistic massage therapist told me to say "I allow my body to heal". That is a very powerful statement when you think about it. I have been trying to live that thought.

The yoga classes are helping to loosen up my tight hip area and bring good energy and blood flow to the area of my body that was affected by the radiation. I also really enjoy the relaxation and positive vibes of the classes.I can sleep better at night without having to make multiple trips to the washroom.

- Six months ago, my PSA at its highest was 48. Normal PSA should be around 1 or 2. Today my PSA is 11. The Doctor was very pleased with this number because she said that most PSA results come down much more slowly over a course of a year and a half. One fellow she knew took two and a half years for his PSA to normalize.
- She also did a digital examination (oh, joy) and noticed that the prostate felt smaller and in good shape. I told her that I was feeling well and peeing well. (After all, peeing is believing.) Love to all.
- Hi Michael, I remember way back you wrote me that after a while one gets used to the sensory overload of burning urine flow. I spoke a prostate cancer survivor I know and he said that occasional irritation can occur for at least a year after radiation.
- I am much relived to be back to my normal peeing self today. Oh, yah. I almost forgot. I still have some corn silk tea that you recommended and it seemed to ease the pain.

- I have not written anything in this column for quite a while. Summer was wonderful. Joan and I biked a lot and I have been active and feeling well. I produced 26 sculptures this year and have felt creative and productive. Gopal and Radha Bello wrote a book called Enlightening Moments and included 20 of my cartoons.
- A year ago I received my diagnosis of prostate cancer. I am much relieved to be on the other side of last fall's radiation treatment. I am also grateful that the after effects of treatment have been minimal. Having to face cancer has altered my perspectives and choices. I only work four days a week now and hardly any evenings. My father's strength was business and work. Much of my practice was modeled after his joy of work and the dedication he had for his clients. I still enjoy my work and I am helping people but I find that I am becoming more and more like my late mother. She was artistic, emotional and loving. I can feel her in me now. I am spending more time doing yoga, drumming and painting my toe nails (please note the spattering of exaggeration and poetic license that may be found herein from time to time).
- A digital examination (no-she did not examine my fingers) revealed that my prostate had shrunk in size and that the left side was soft, but that the right side was still a little firm. She felt that all was well and scheduled my next examination for April, 2012.

- I can watch an entire movie without having to get up and pee. I feel energetic and healthy most of the time. I will continue to live my life with love and joy and have faith that my path will unfold as it is meant to for infinity and beyond.

Michael, thank you, may your writing flow like a man with a healthy prostate…
Hurry up we need the pens……
For more information on Allan see www.allanhirsh.com

About The Author

The health system is something Michael knows intimately. He worked with several health systems for over twenty five years in North America, Europe and Australia.

Like the vast majority of people in the field his goal was to help improve the way healthcare was delivered to ultimately help make more people well. Michael and his wife Elizabeth worked with hospitals, clinics, research agencies, charities and health centres to try to help them balance the competing demands for resources.

They helped health care providers get more resources for their work, they obtained more money for research, and set up systems that were more responsive to patient needs. One example being a cardiovascular surgery urgency system which reduced deaths of patients on waiting lists. They devised software to help healthcare managers better allocate resources. This helped them understand health information and the systems that deliver services to cancer patients.

For the three years leading up to this book being published, Michael has been a patient with often daily contact with health professionals because of his cancer diagnosis. He says that seeing health care from the other side of the fence has been both rewarding and eye opening. Michael's respect for most of the health care providers of all stripes has not diminished.

While Michael was part of the health system in some ways he led a double life. In his spare time Michael worked to understand healing from non-traditional angles. Michael became aware that science was unable to adequately understand alternative healing and as a result tended to write it off even when there were interesting findings.

His work in the field of meditation is well known. His first book on the subject, “Meditation Good Medicine” was written in 1999 to help stimulate more scholarly research into this method of reducing stress and promoting wellness. This book was followed by “Meditation for Enduring Happiness” in 2011, a book to help all of us understand meditation and the science behind it. The book leads the reader through 42 meditations to help the reader understand and achieve enduring happiness.

After proving the effectiveness of meditation Michael realized that there are many other areas with promising results that need a magnifying glass applied to them in the same way. Importantly, once diagnosed with cancer he started to look very closely at all aspects of cancer. That initiated the impetus for this book.

In addition to being a person diagnosed with cancer, Michael has a background as a scientist with academic training in health science, psychology and biology as well as environmental studies. He has researched many areas that contribute to cancer, from environmental carcinogens to the psychology of stress. As such he has the important point of view of a well trained insider with patient experience.

Michael wrote this book to share his discoveries with others in hopes that all who read this book can become empowered, regain their health and beat the odds against cancer.

Michael can be contacted through the publisher or through his personal website (www.MichaeljMcCartney.com). Other books by the author follow.

Books By Michael J. McCartney

Cancer_Beating the Odds 2012

Meditation for Enduring Happiness 2011

Meditation Good Medicine 1999

The books are available on Amazon and in bookstores or they can be ordered directly from Archangel Publications.

4980B Prince Edward Road One

RR2, Consecon,

Ontario, Canada

K0K1T0

Look for upcoming books at

www.Archangel-Books.com

or contact the publisher

Liz Fleming

LizArchangelPublications@gmail.com